PAULA
BAYSINGER
MORHARDT

Is This My Grandma?

ILLUSTRATIONS BY
KIM HANZO

TEACUP PRESS

Copyright © 2021 by Paula Baysinger Morhardt

All rights reserved. Published in the United States by Teacup Press, an imprint of Fox Pointe Publishing, LLP. No part of this book may be reproduced in any form or by any electronic or mechanical means, including information storage and retrieval systems, without permission in writing from the publisher.

www.teacup-press.com • www.foxpointepublishing.com/author-paula-morhardt

Library of Congress Cataloging-in-Publication Data
Morhardt, Paula Baysinger, author.
Eckman, Raven, editor.
Hanzo, Kim, illustrator.
Hudson, Becca, designer.

Is This My Grandma? / Paula Baysinger Morhardt. – First edition.

Summary: When two young children visit their grandmother in the hospital, the older sibling helps the younger sibling understand what is happening.

ISBN 979-8-9998837-9-7 (hardcover) / 978-1-952567-85-8 (softcover)
[1. Grandparents – Fiction. 2. Diseases, Illnesses, & Injuries – Fiction. 3. New Experience – Fiction. 4. Emotions & Feelings – Fiction.]

Library of Congress Control Number: 2 0 2 1 9 0 9 4 1 9

2nd printing October 2025

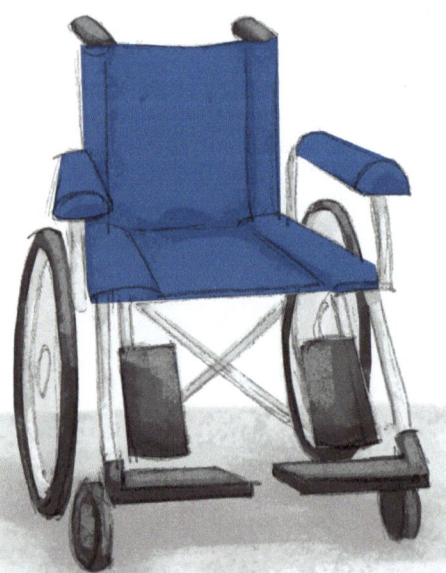

To Abby, Brianna, Matthew, Benjamin, and especially Caleb, who was once that little boy who said "I scared."

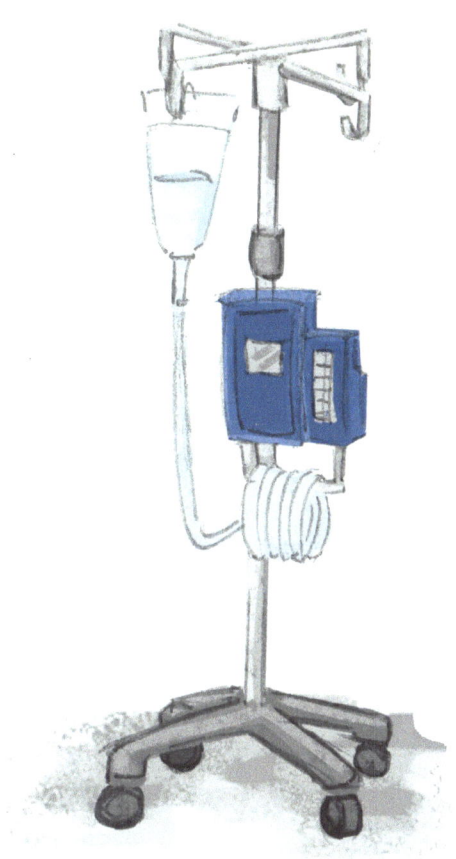

Mama told my brother and I
we were going to visit Grandma.

I love Grandma!

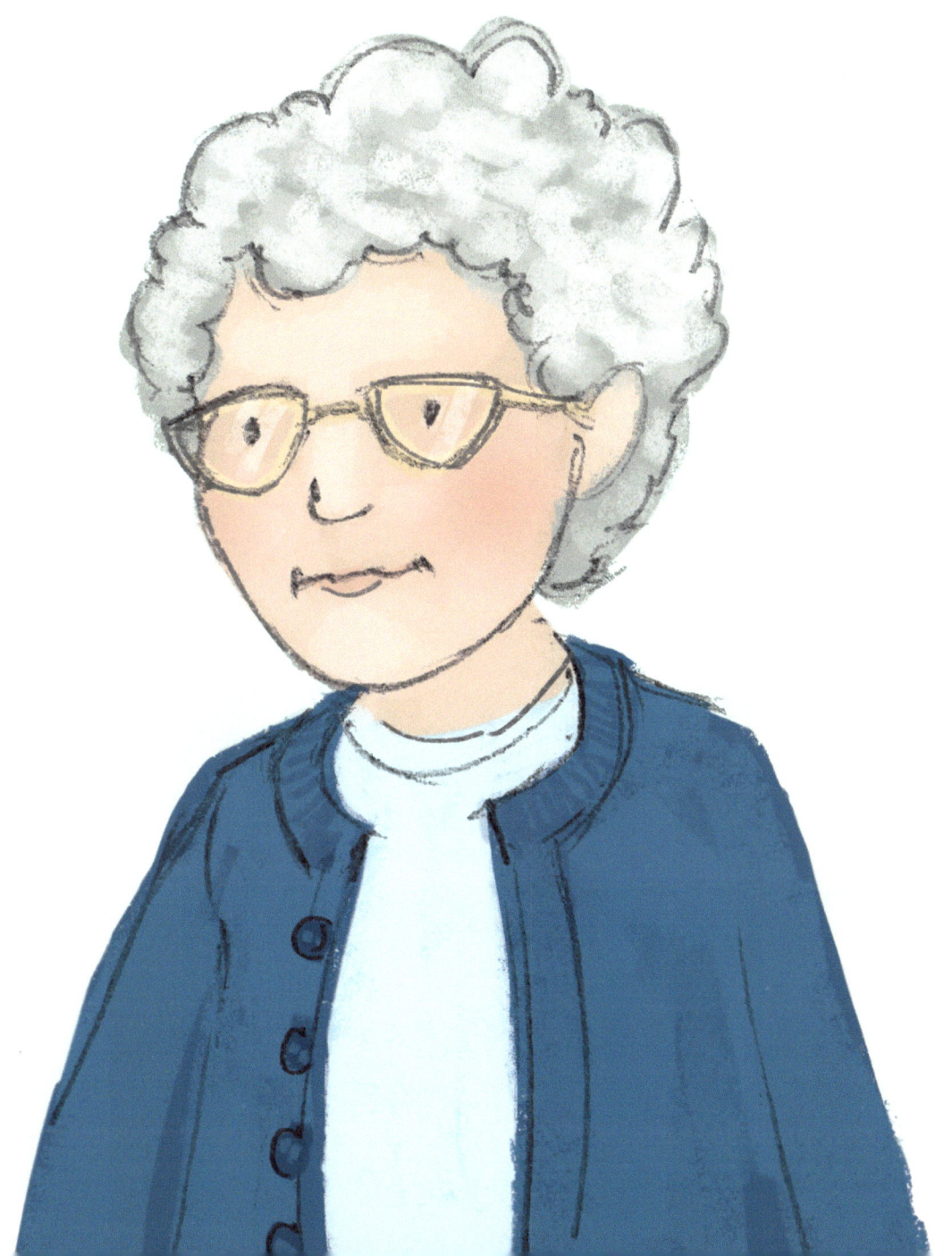

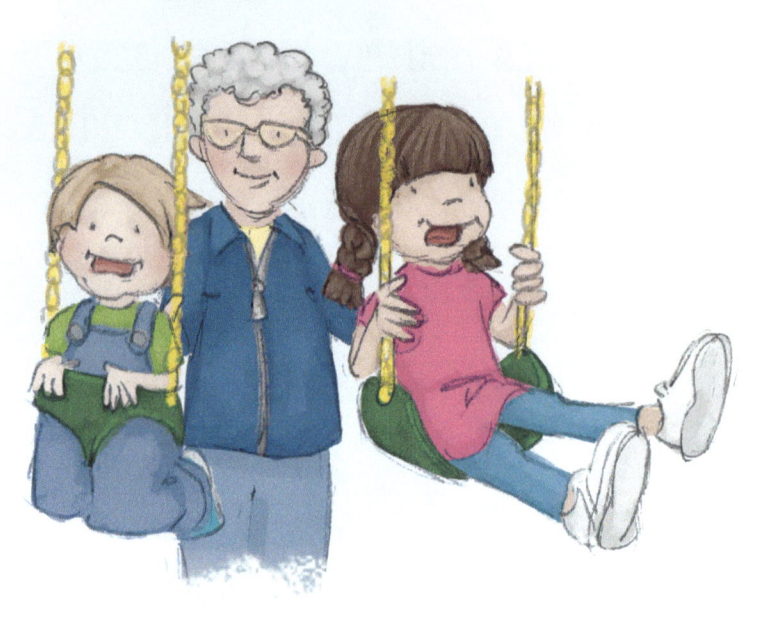

She pushes me on the swing and plays with my little brother in the sandbox.

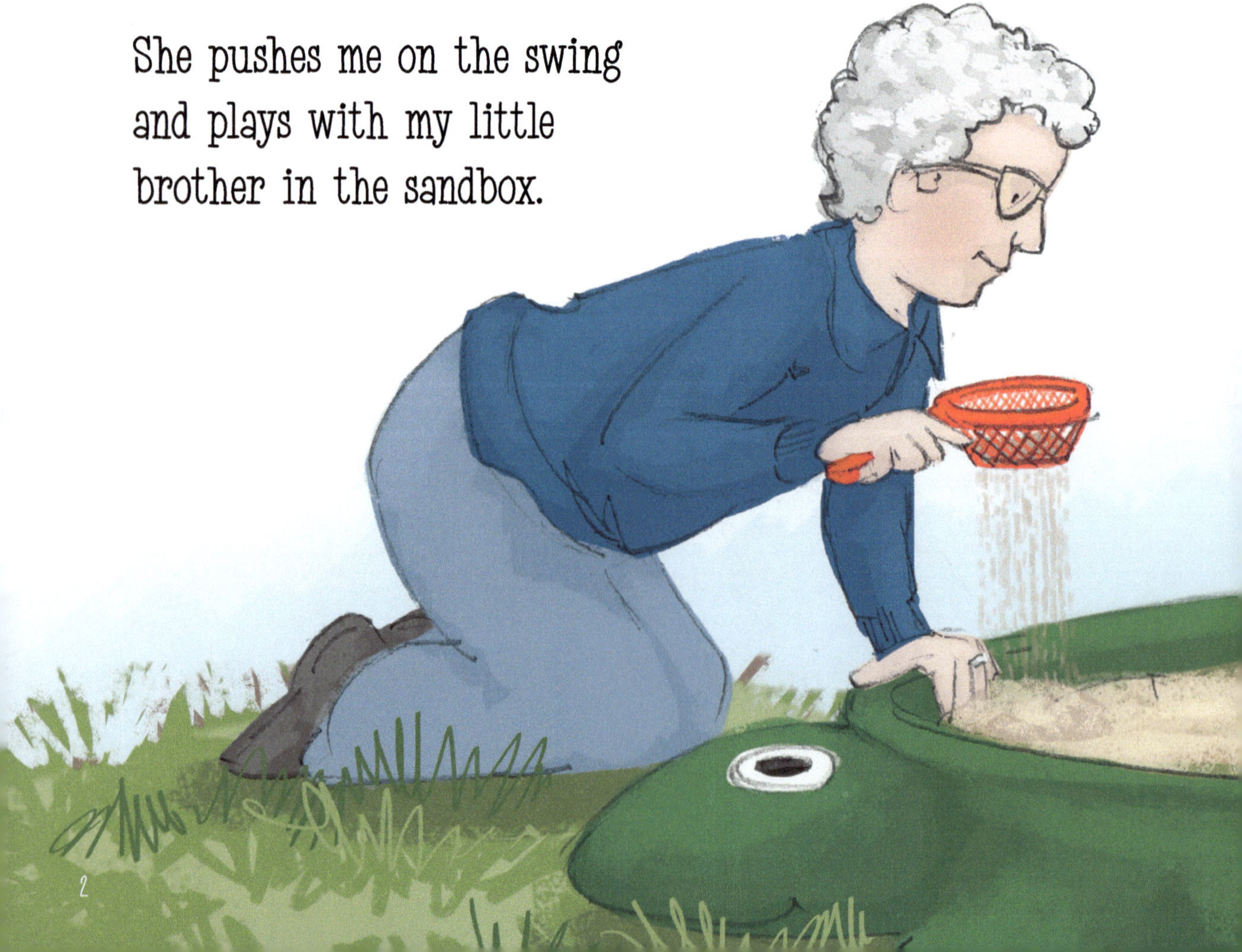

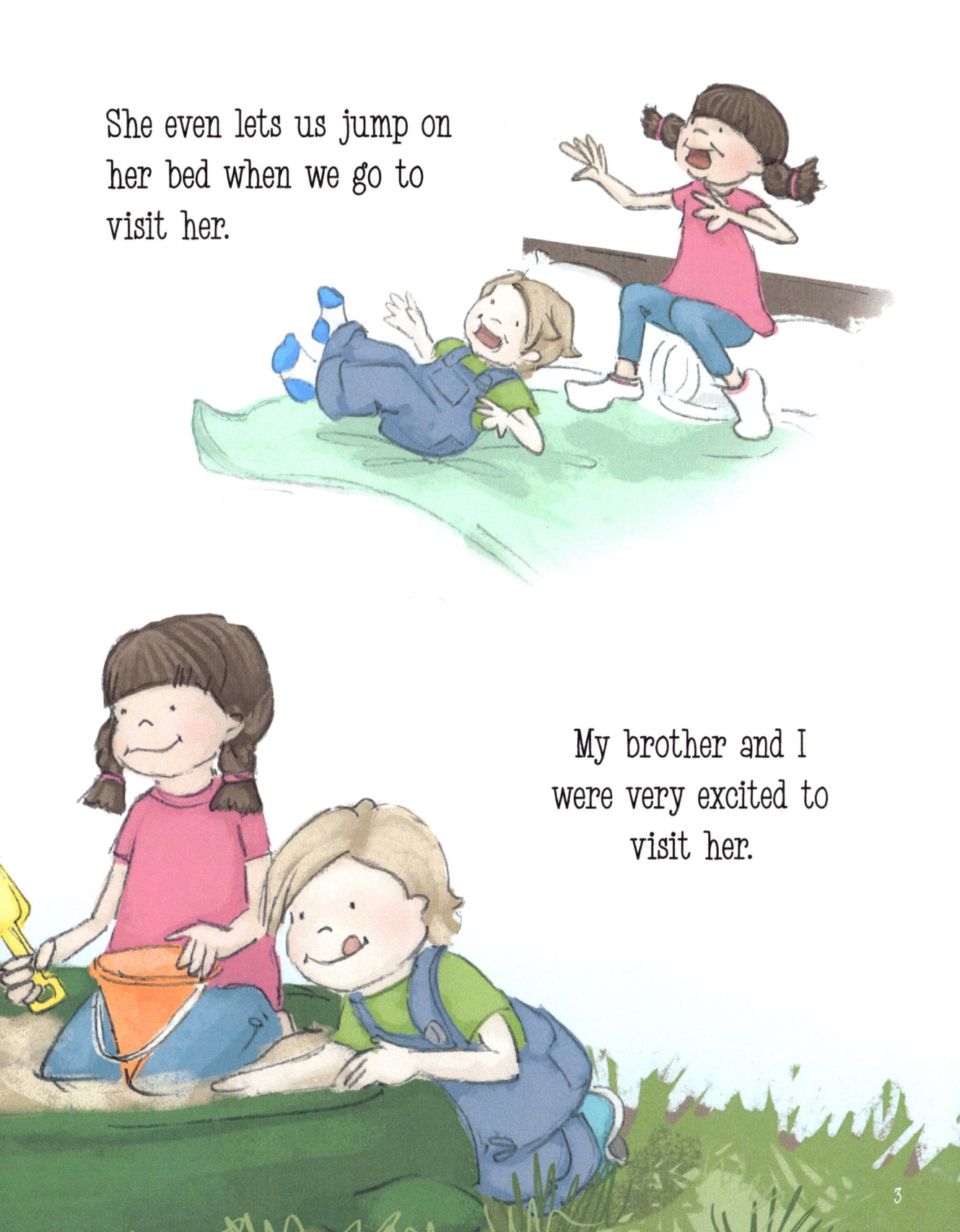

She even lets us jump on her bed when we go to visit her.

My brother and I were very excited to visit her.

But...Mama didn't drive to Grandma's house. She drove to a big building made of red brick with lots of windows.

I remembered the building from when Grandma was sick before.

I looked at my brother in his car seat. "This is a hospital," I said.

He looked scared, so I grabbed his hand.

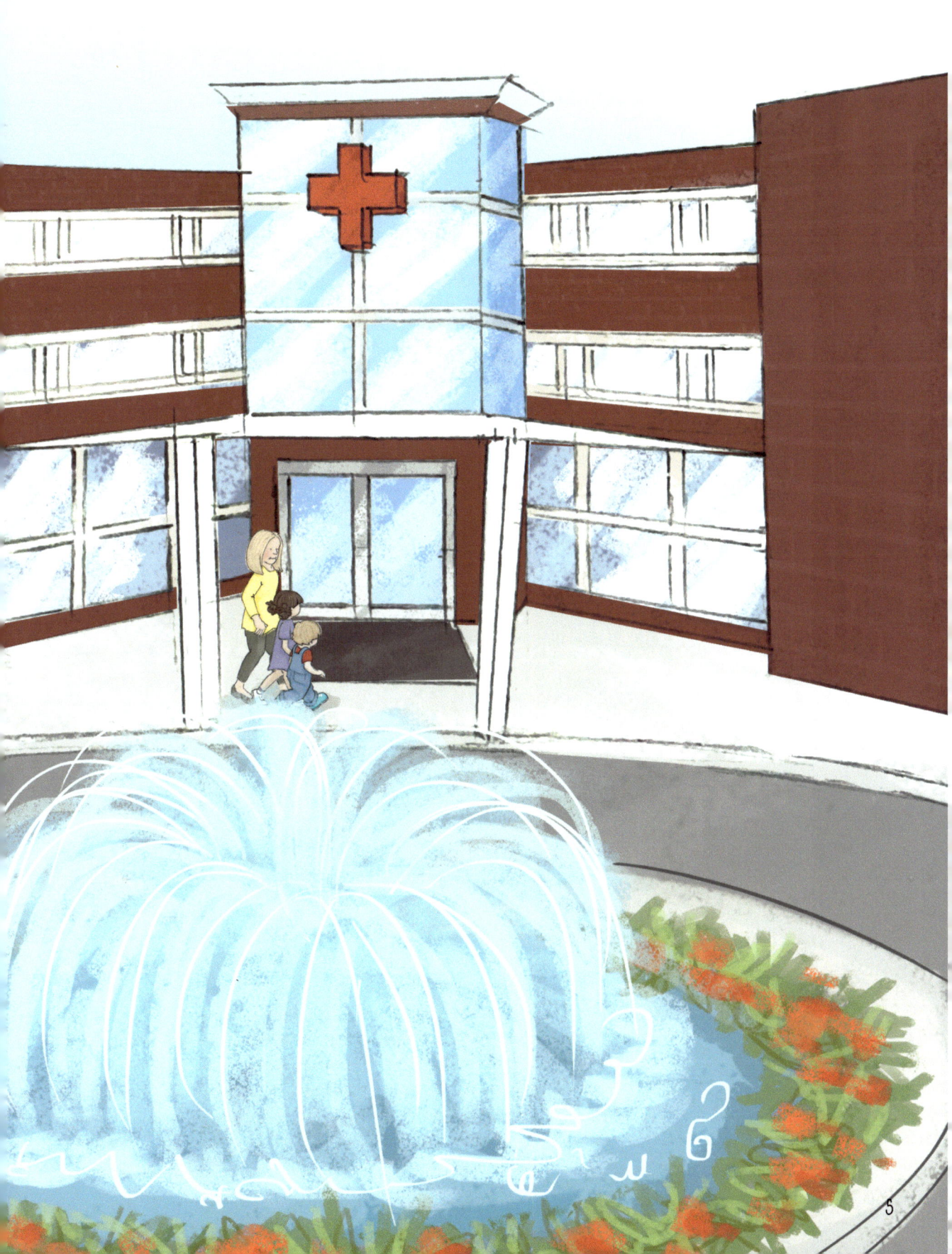

When we walked into the building,
we went into a little room called an elevator.

There were buttons with numbers on them.

Mama let my brother push
the number three button.

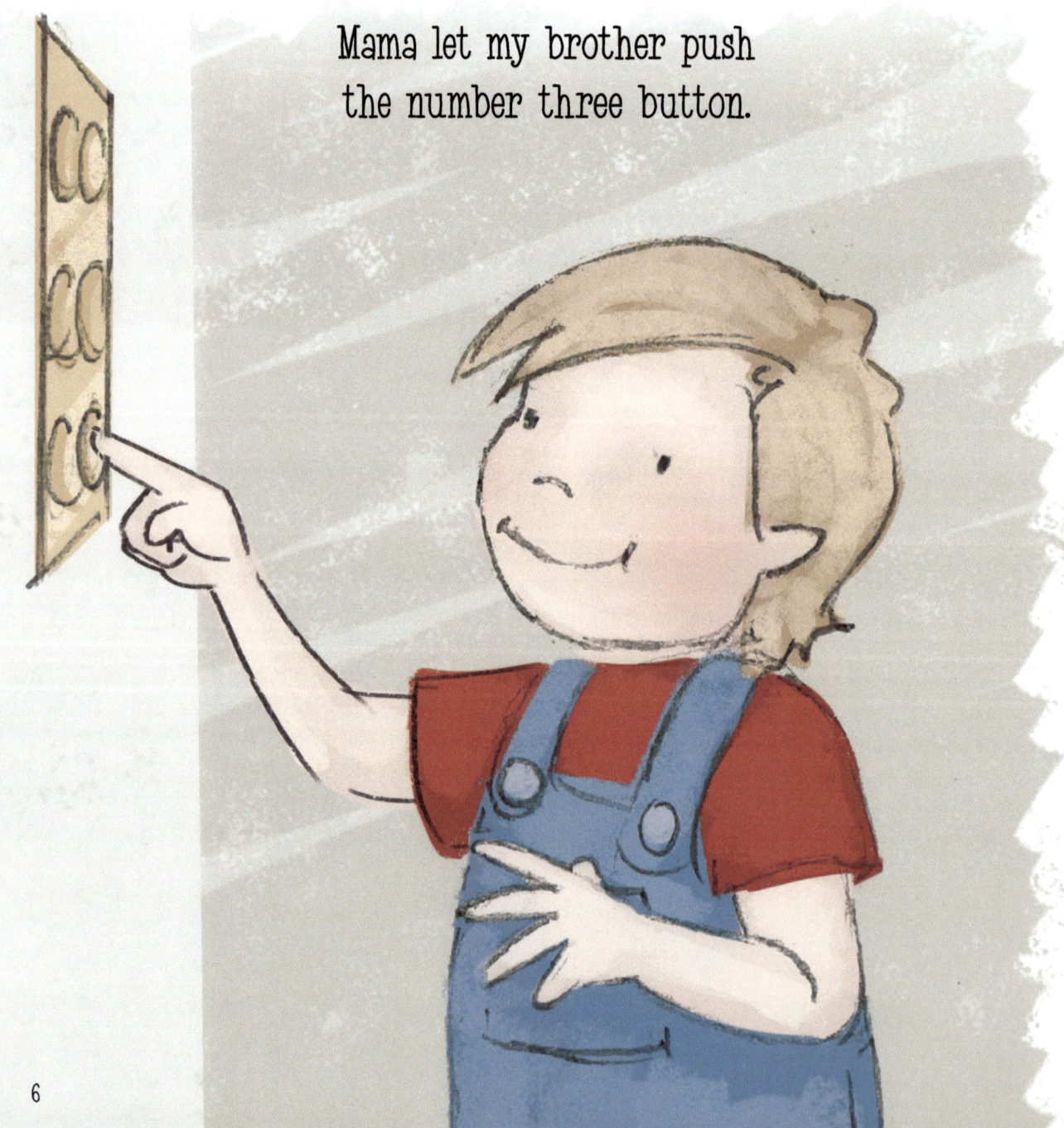

I laughed with Mama because my brother's eyes got really big when the elevator doors closed, but then he giggled when the elevator suddenly went up.

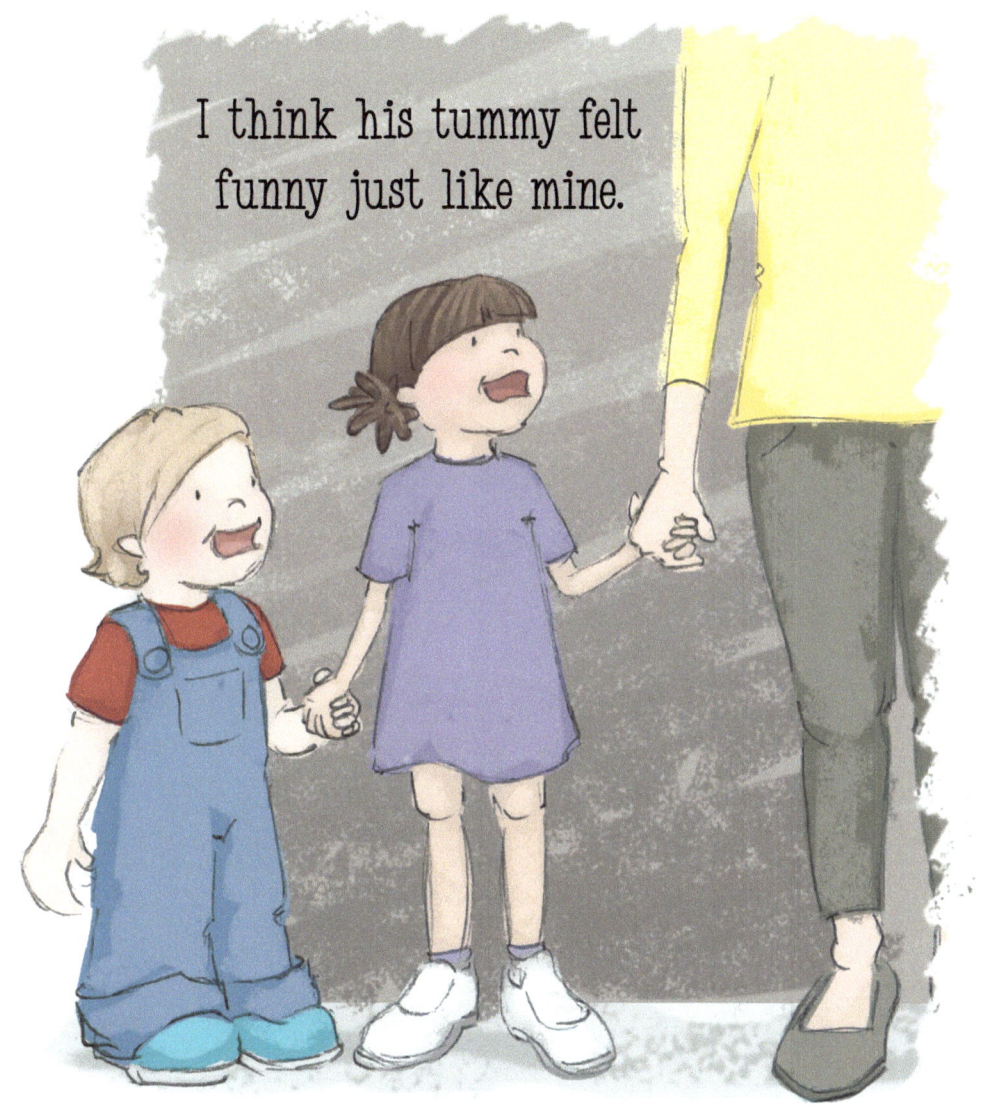

I think his tummy felt funny just like mine.

I kept holding his hand as the elevator doors opened again; Mama took my other hand.

We walked down a long hallway with lots of doors.
There were doctors and nurses everywhere,
and a loud voice was talking from the ceiling.

I remembered the voice from before, so I wasn't scared.

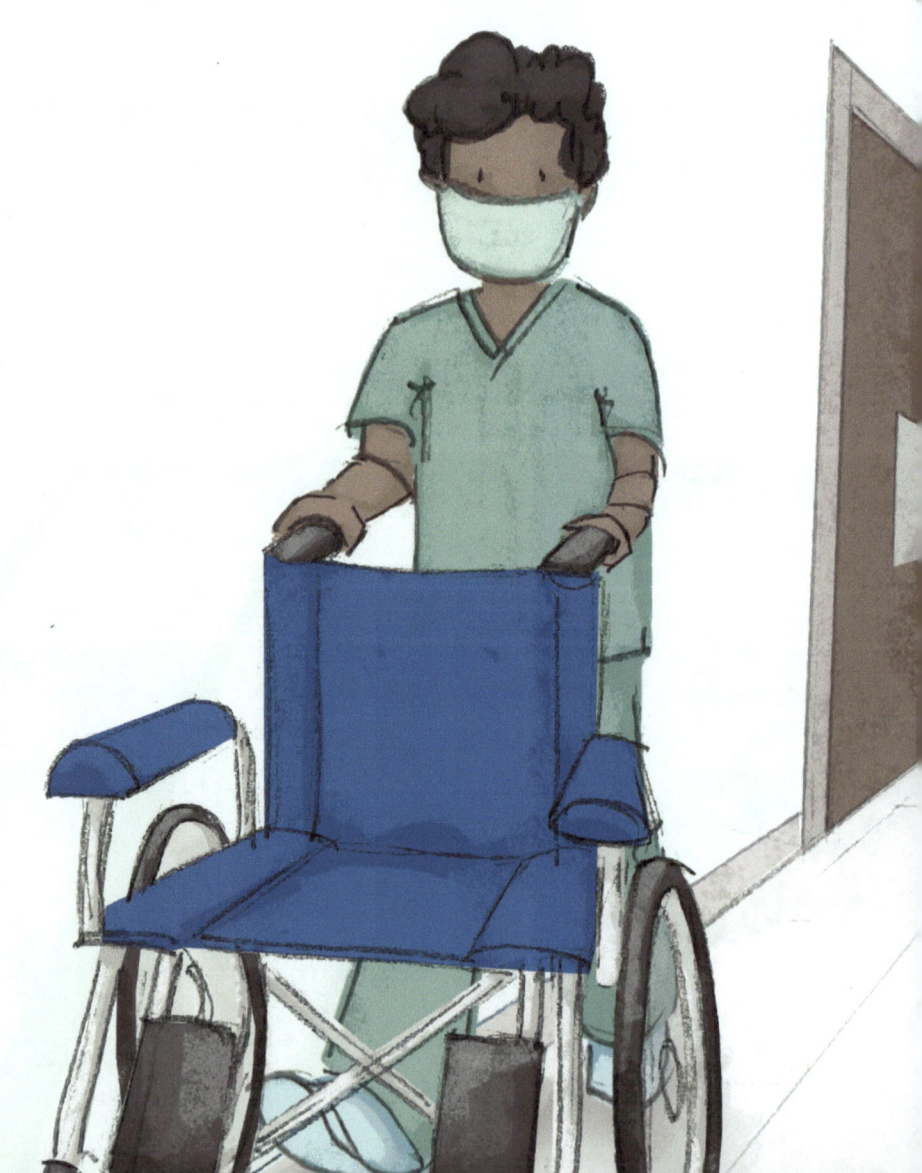

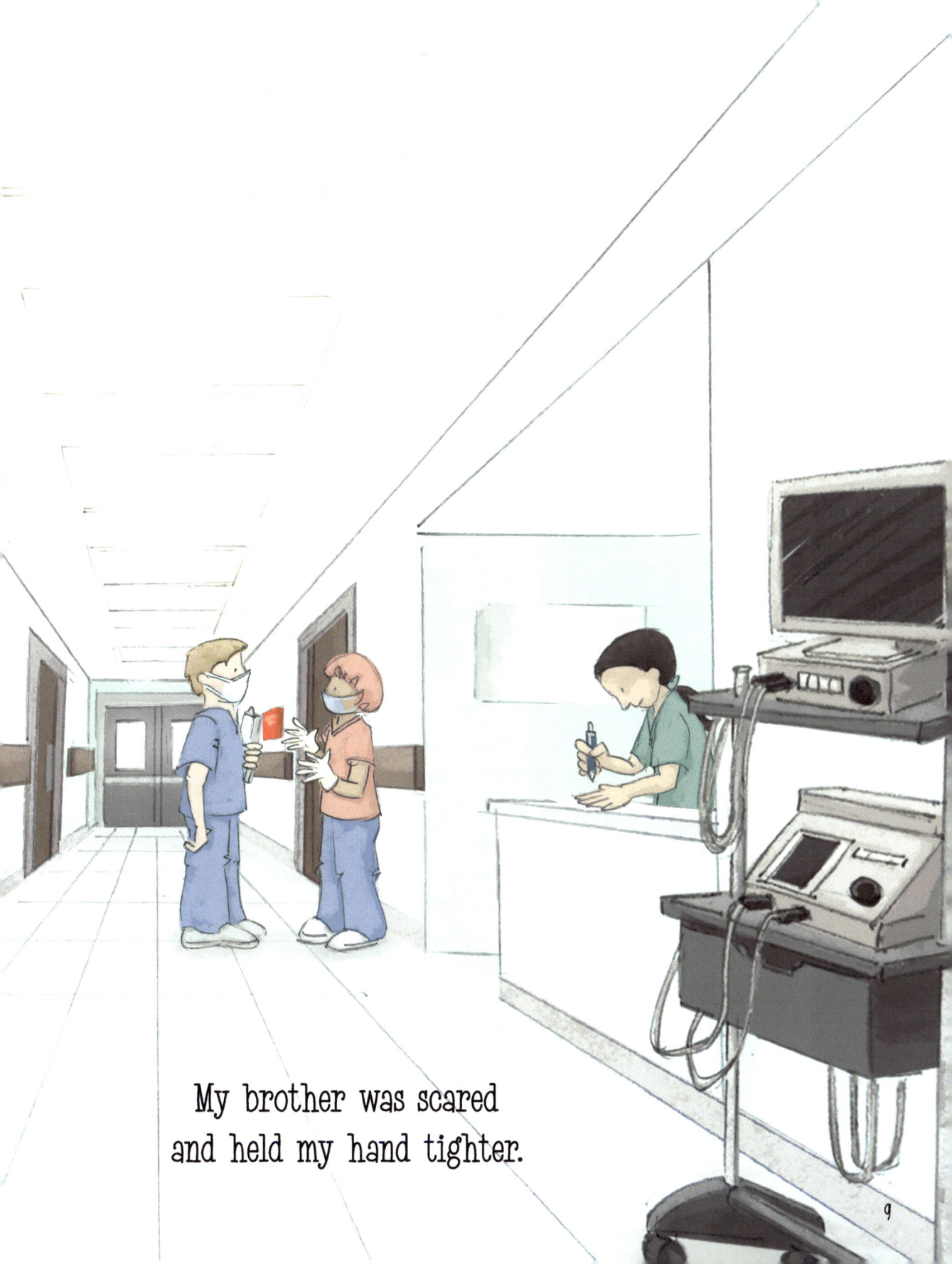
My brother was scared and held my hand tighter.

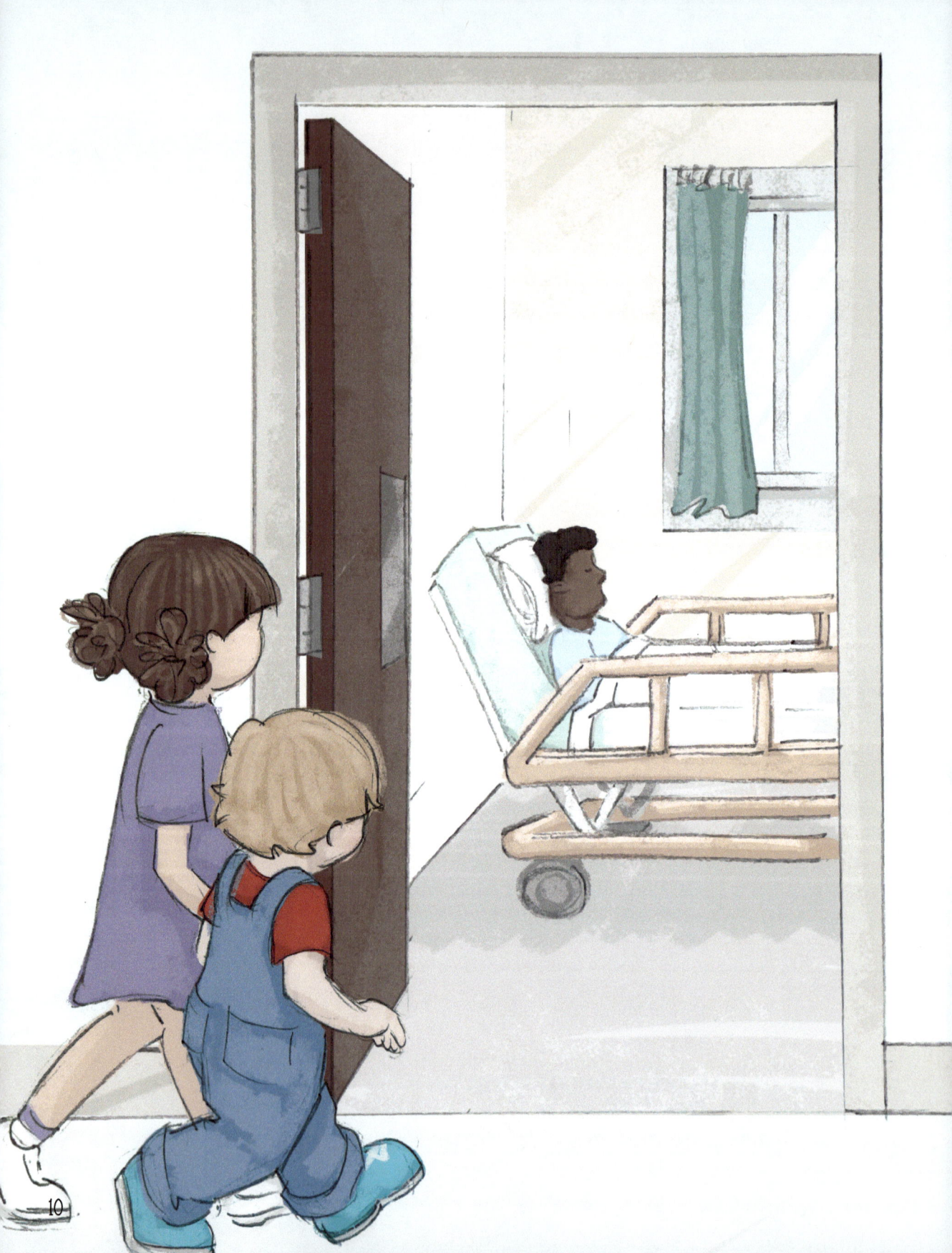

When I looked in the open doors, there were funny looking beds in the rooms. They had long metal rails on them, and the people could sit up with the bed.

Some of the beds had people in them, and they were wearing their pajamas!

I said to my brother, "I wonder if we could wear our pajamas when we visit Grandma here!"

He smiled a little, which made me feel good.

He looked scared, so I grabbed his hand.

My brother whispered to me, "I scared," so I smiled at him, trying to be brave, and told him there was nothing to be scared of.

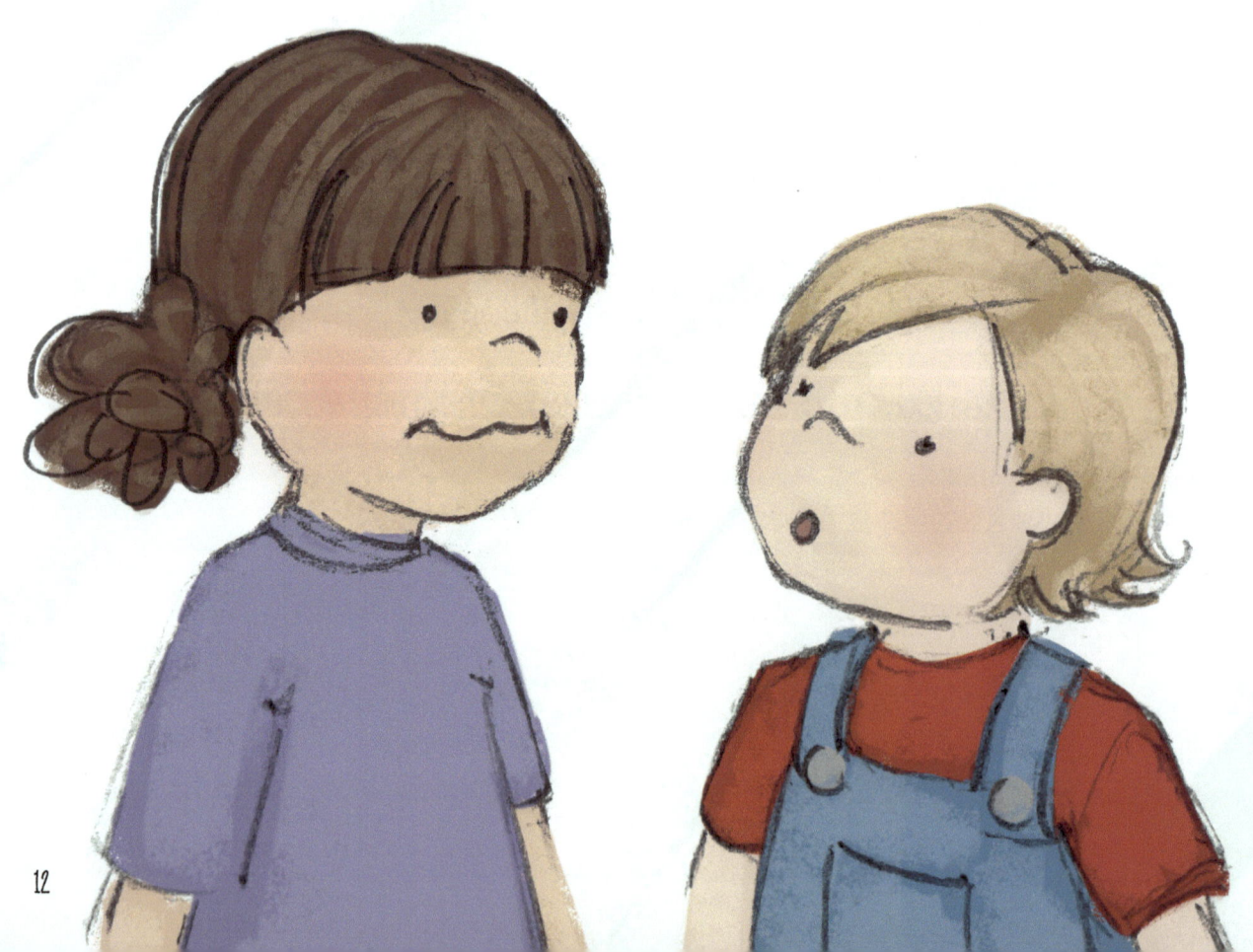

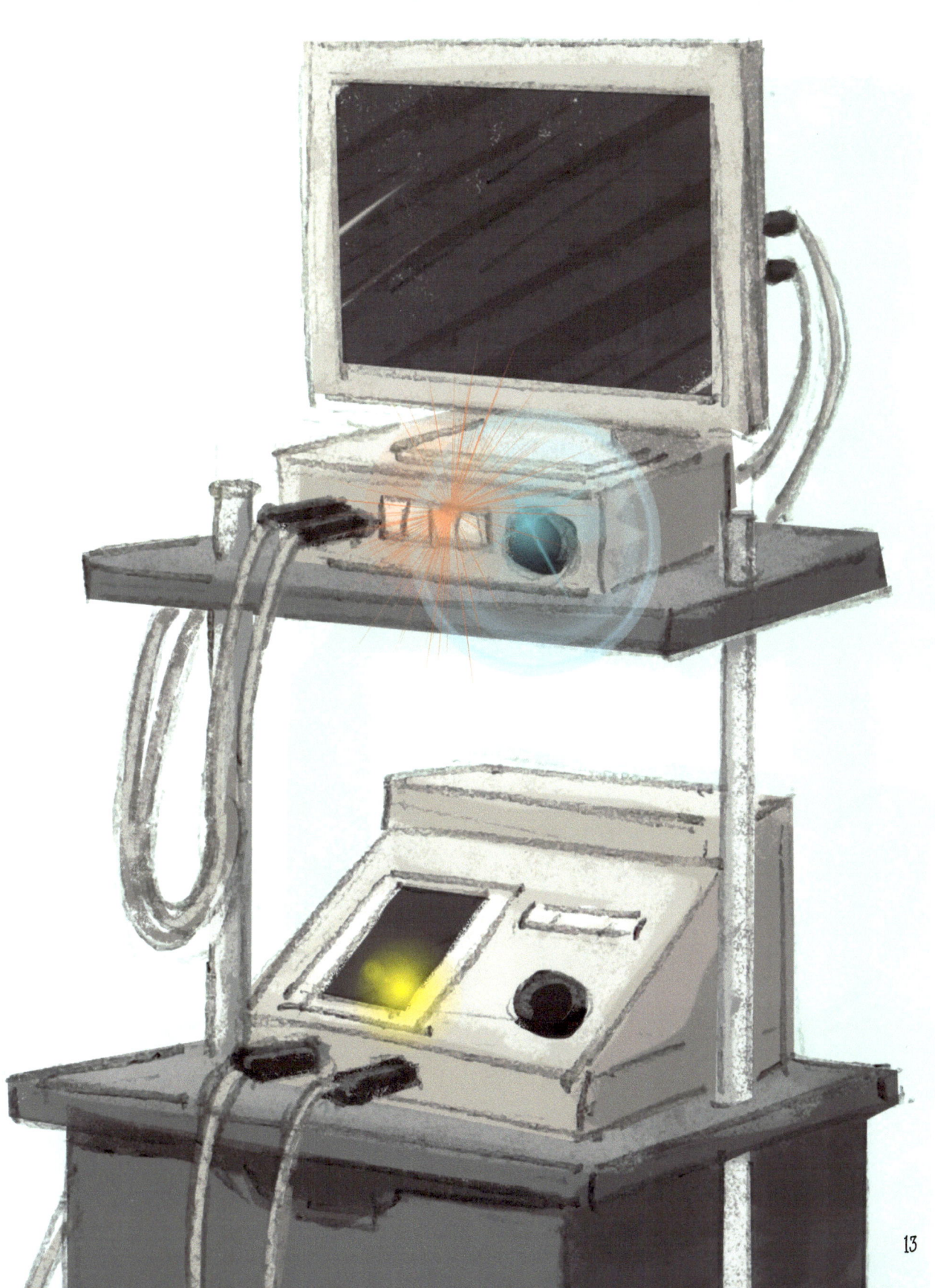

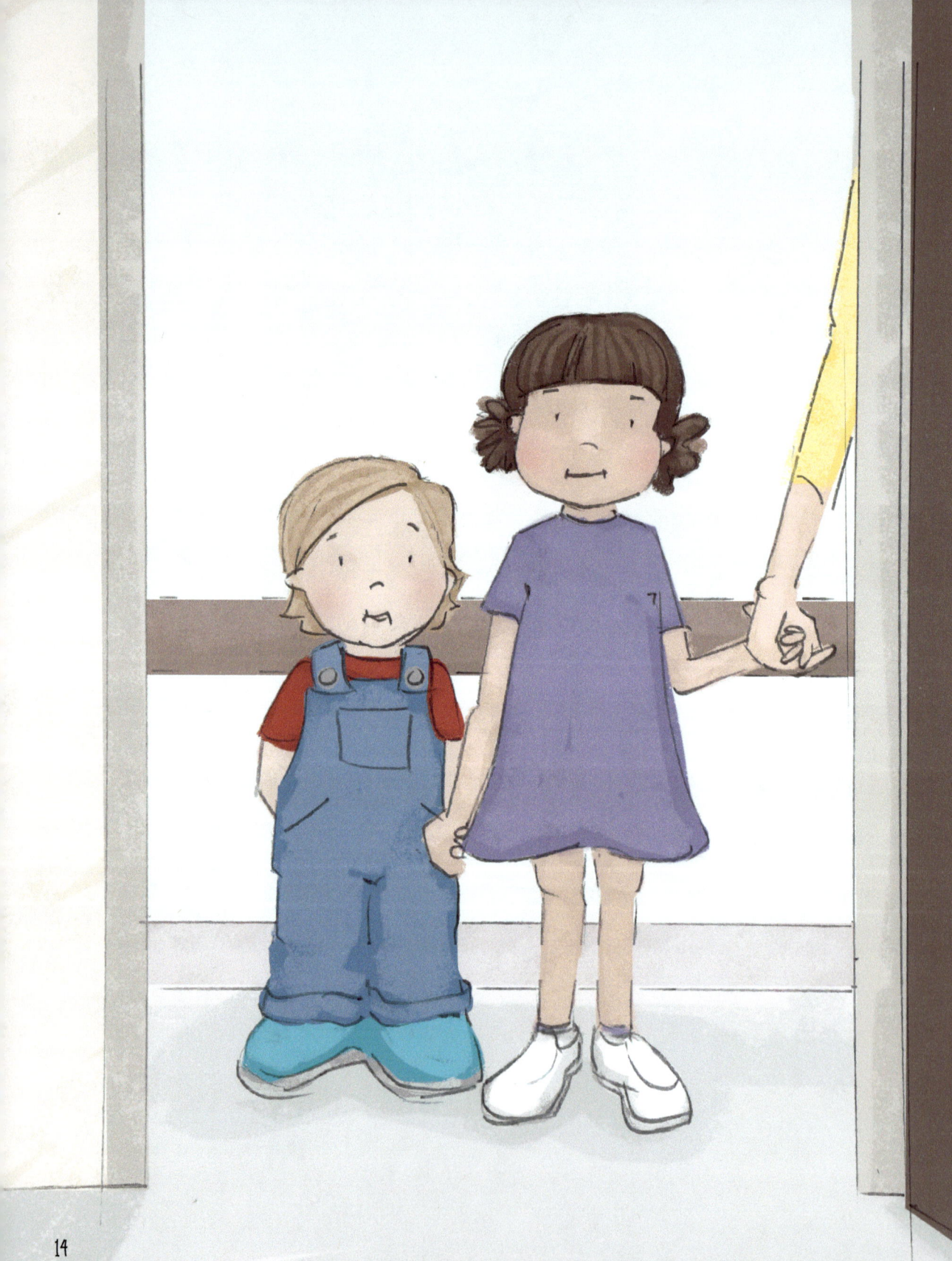

We stopped at one of the doors near
the end of the hallway and Mama said
this was where Grandma was.

My little brother didn't understand.
I knew he thought Grandma only lived at her
house, just like I had thought when I was his age.

He didn't know that sometimes she had to stay at
the hospital to get better when she was sick.

I held his hand very carefully so he wouldn't run
away when we stepped into the room.

"I scared," he said again, and Mama gave him a hug
before leading us into the room.

I took a step forward, to be brave, but stopped.

Grandma had tubes in her nose, and another tube stuck in her arm. There was a machine with blinking lights, and it was making a loud hissing noise.

I knew I had seen all this before, but it was very loud. I was a little bit scared again.

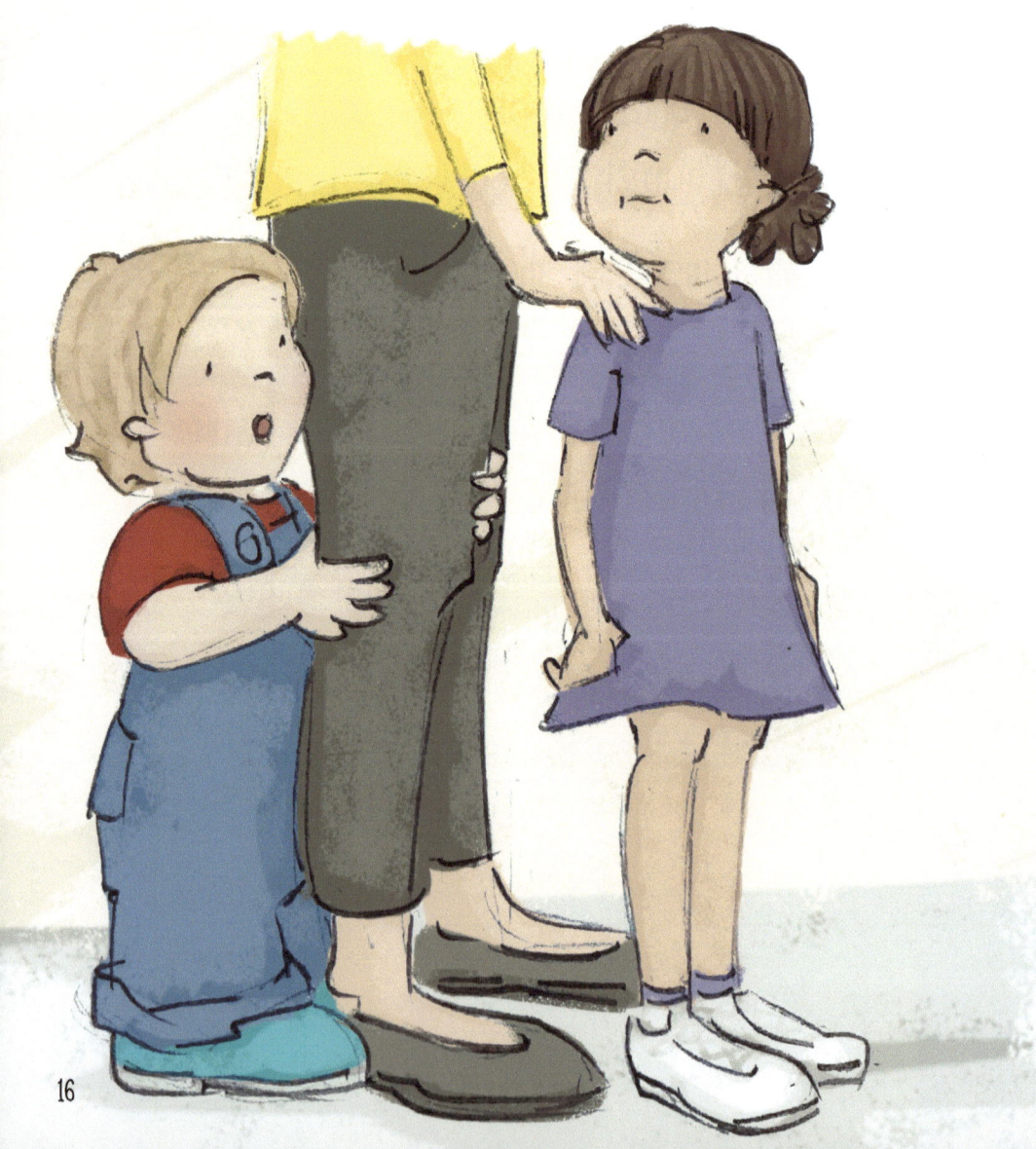

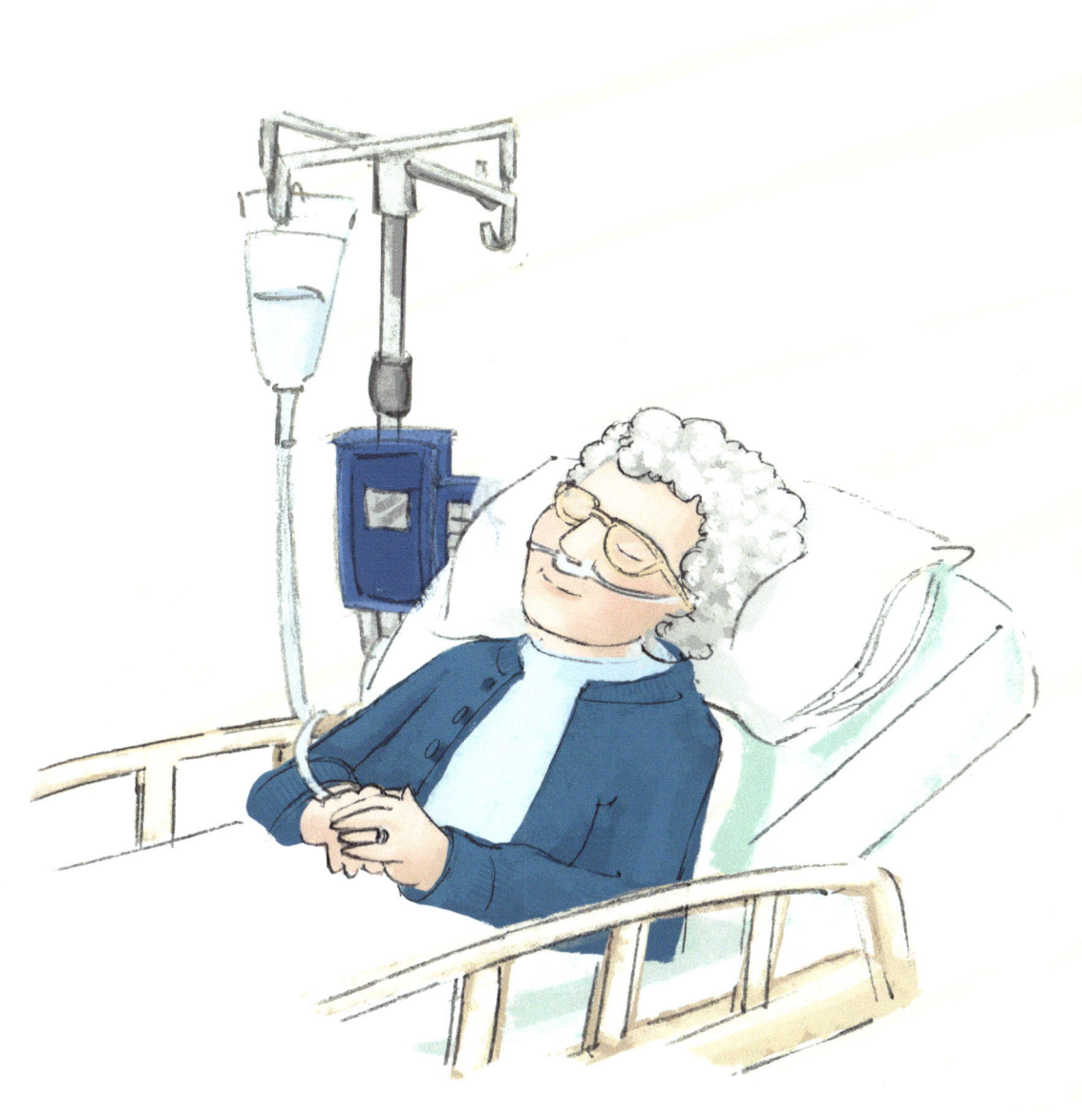

My brother cried, "NOT Grandma!"
and ran to hide behind Mama.

I remembered that I had to be brave because this WAS Grandma.

I walked up to the bed and patted Grandma's hand.

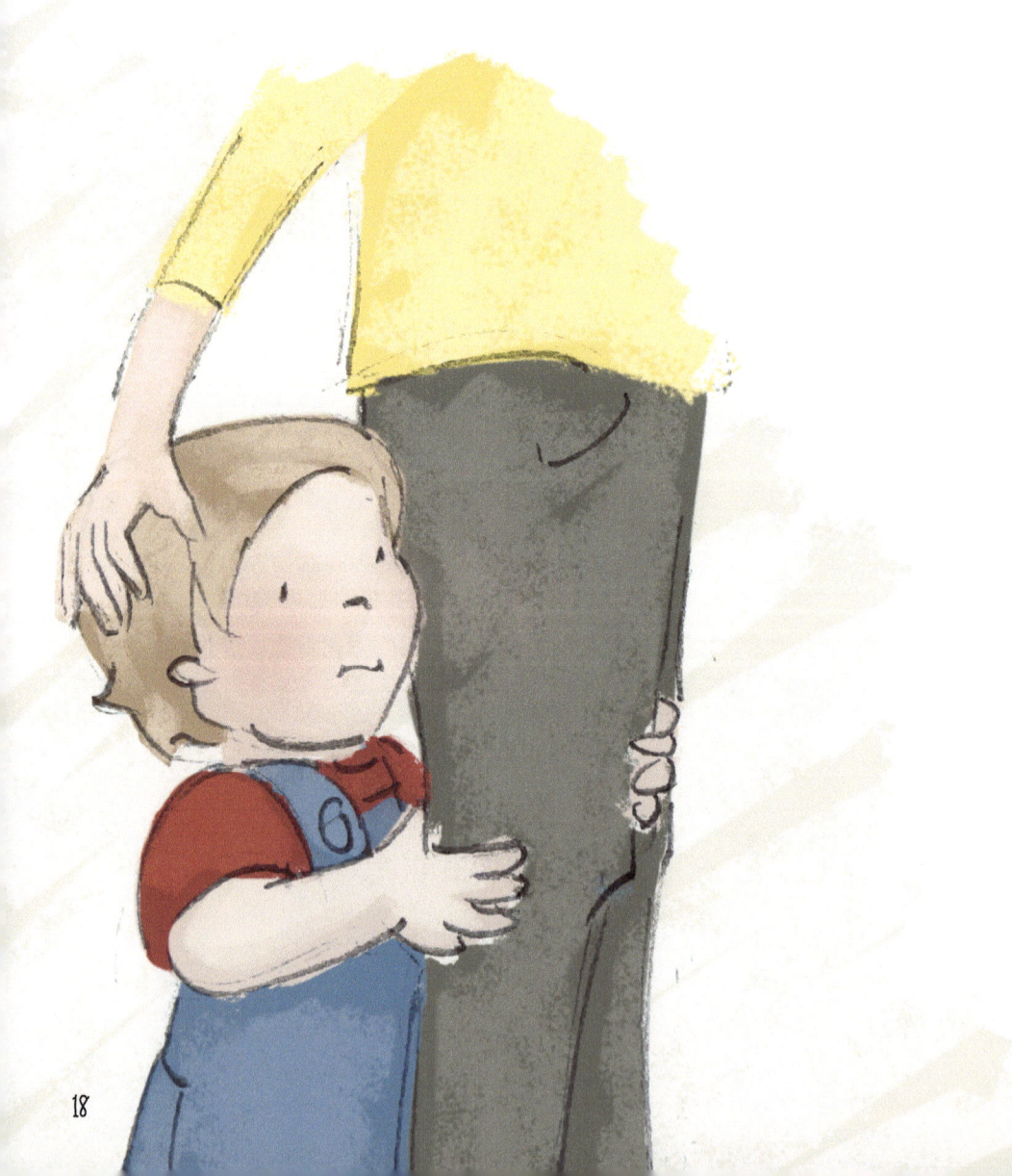

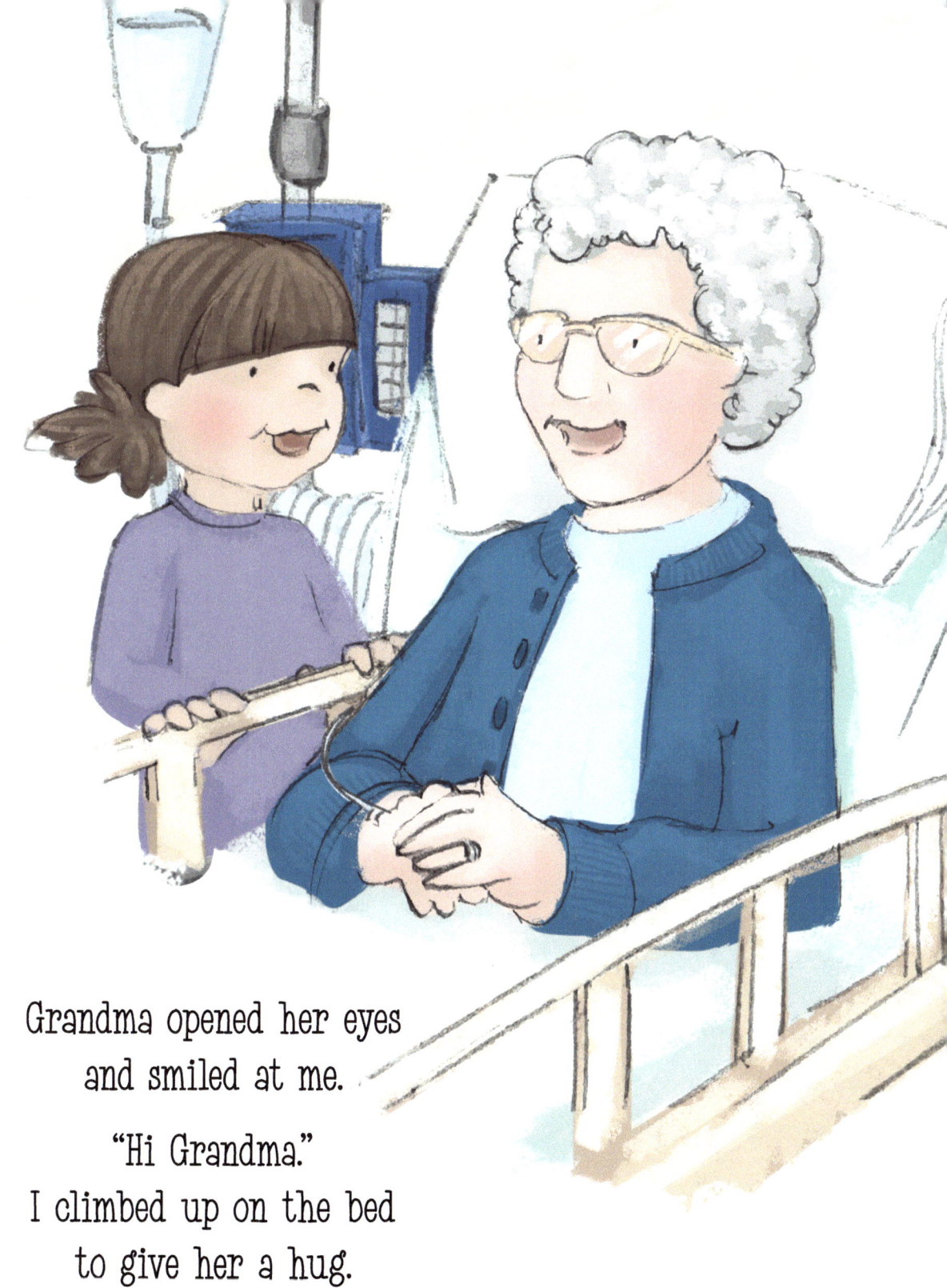

Grandma opened her eyes
and smiled at me.

"Hi Grandma."
I climbed up on the bed
to give her a hug.

I looked back at my brother and could tell he was still scared, so I left Grandma's bedside to go talk to him.

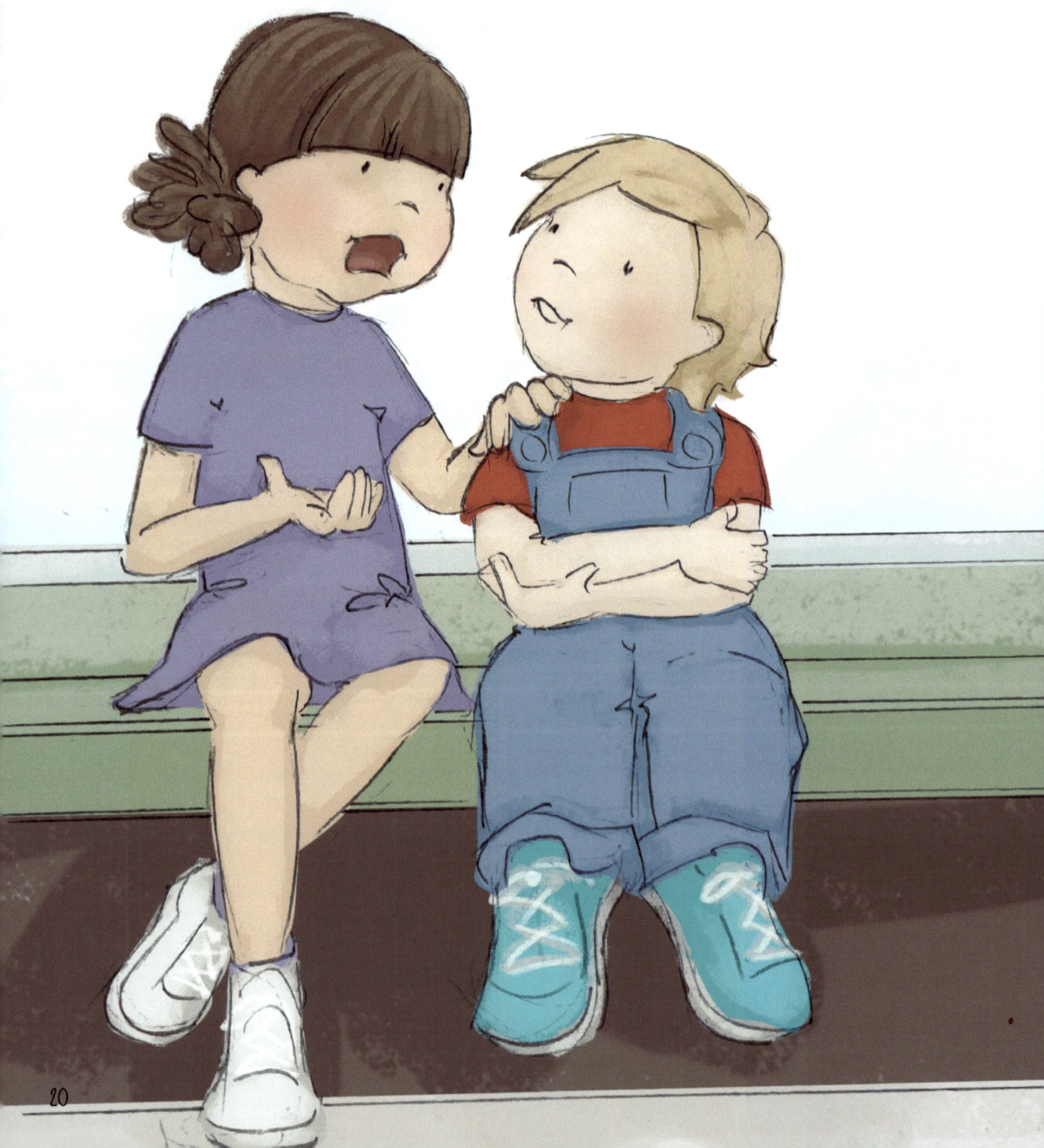

I told him that sometimes Grandma had to come and stay at the hospital so the doctors could make her feel better.

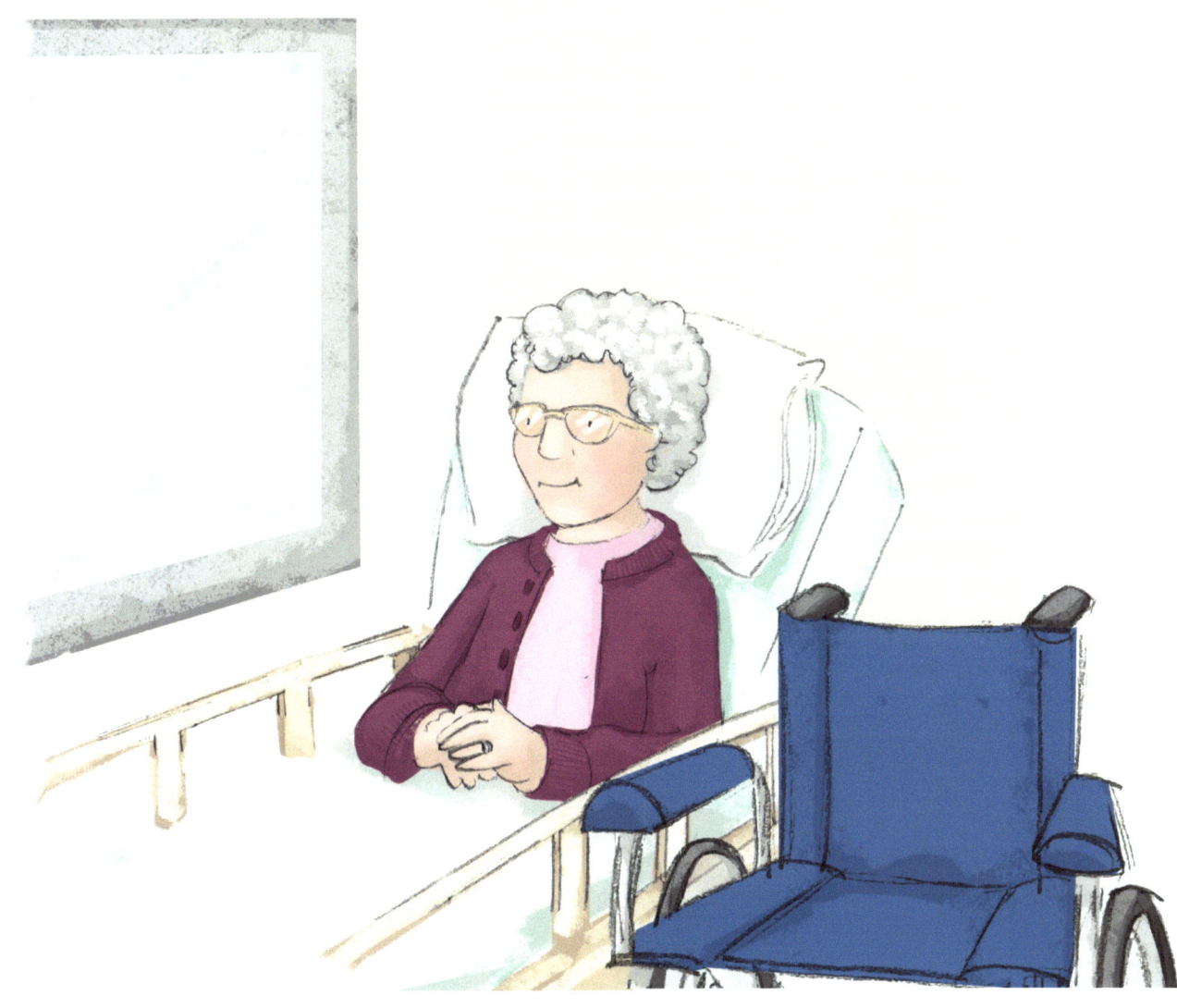

He didn't understand because he didn't remember Grandma ever being sick. He was too little to remember.

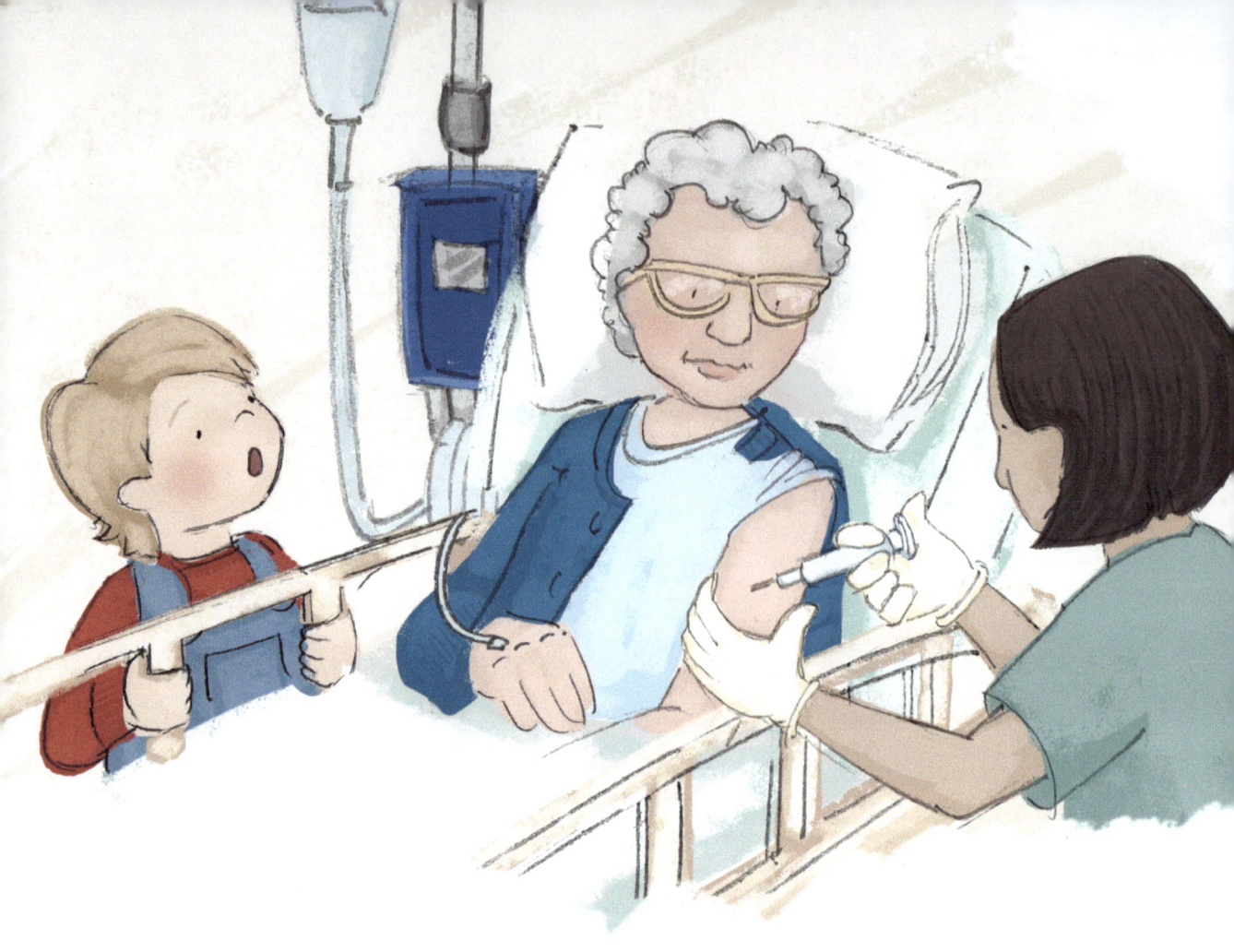

Just then, a nurse came in with a needle and gave Grandma a shot.

My brother was very scared of shots, but when the nurse smiled at him, he smiled back.

The nurse left and came back with a funny thing that had four feet and a bar; it was called a "walker".

It was to help Grandma walk.

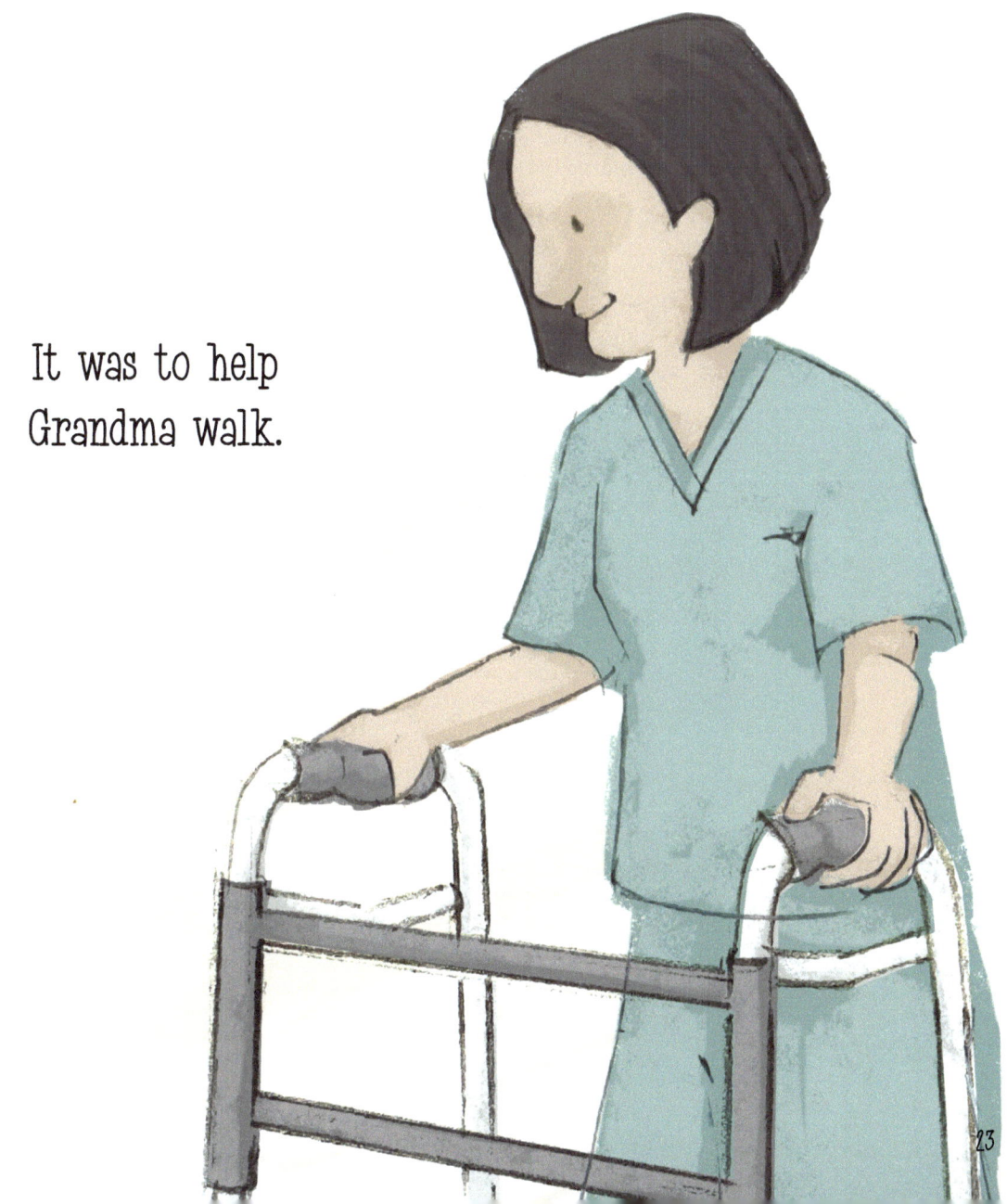

The nurse and Mama helped Grandma get out of bed and stand up. She had a bandage on her leg from her toes to up under her nightgown!

Grandma cried a little bit when they stood her up, and that made me sad—Grandma doesn't cry!

My little brother made a small noise in his throat, so I went and took his hand.

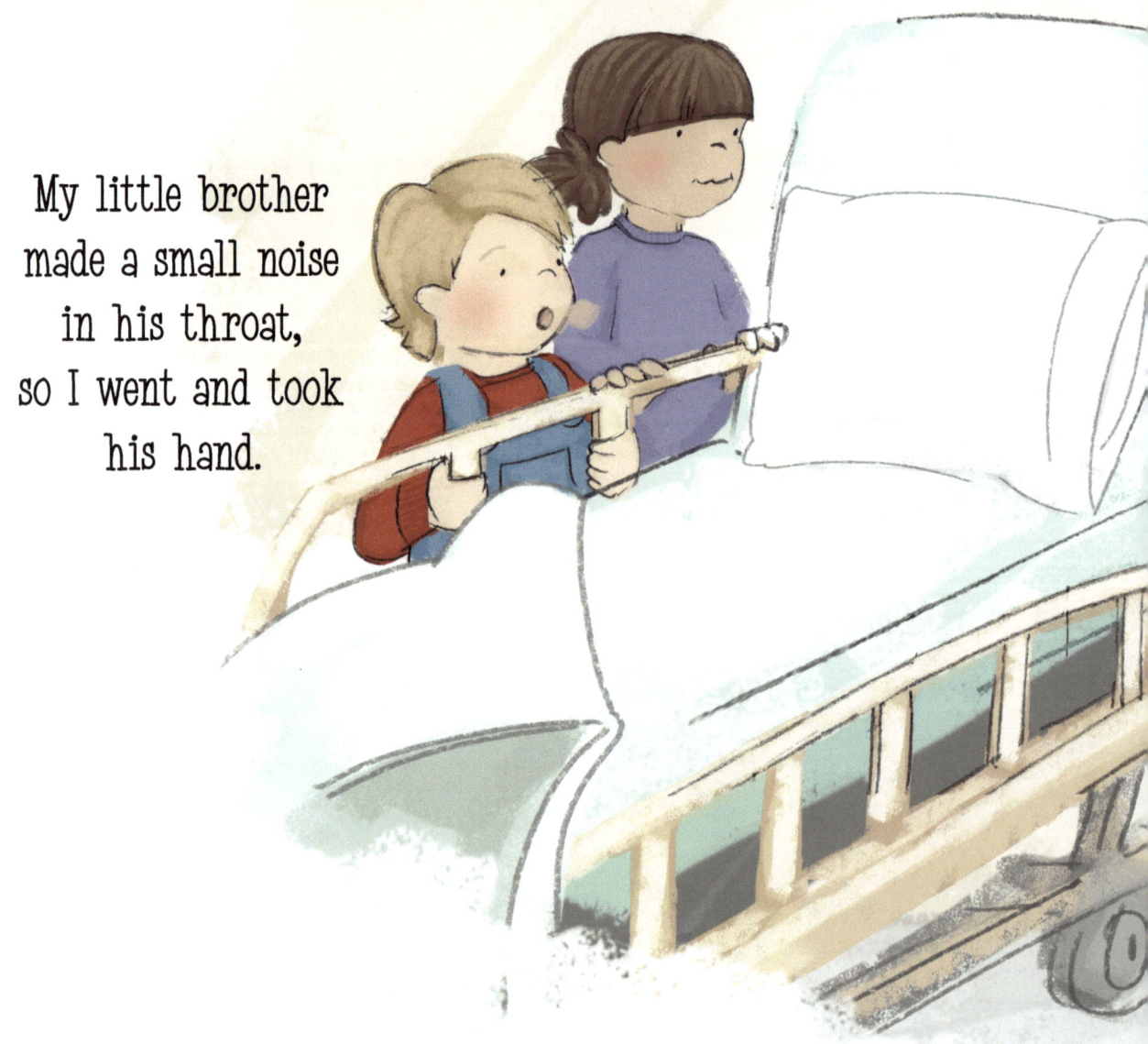

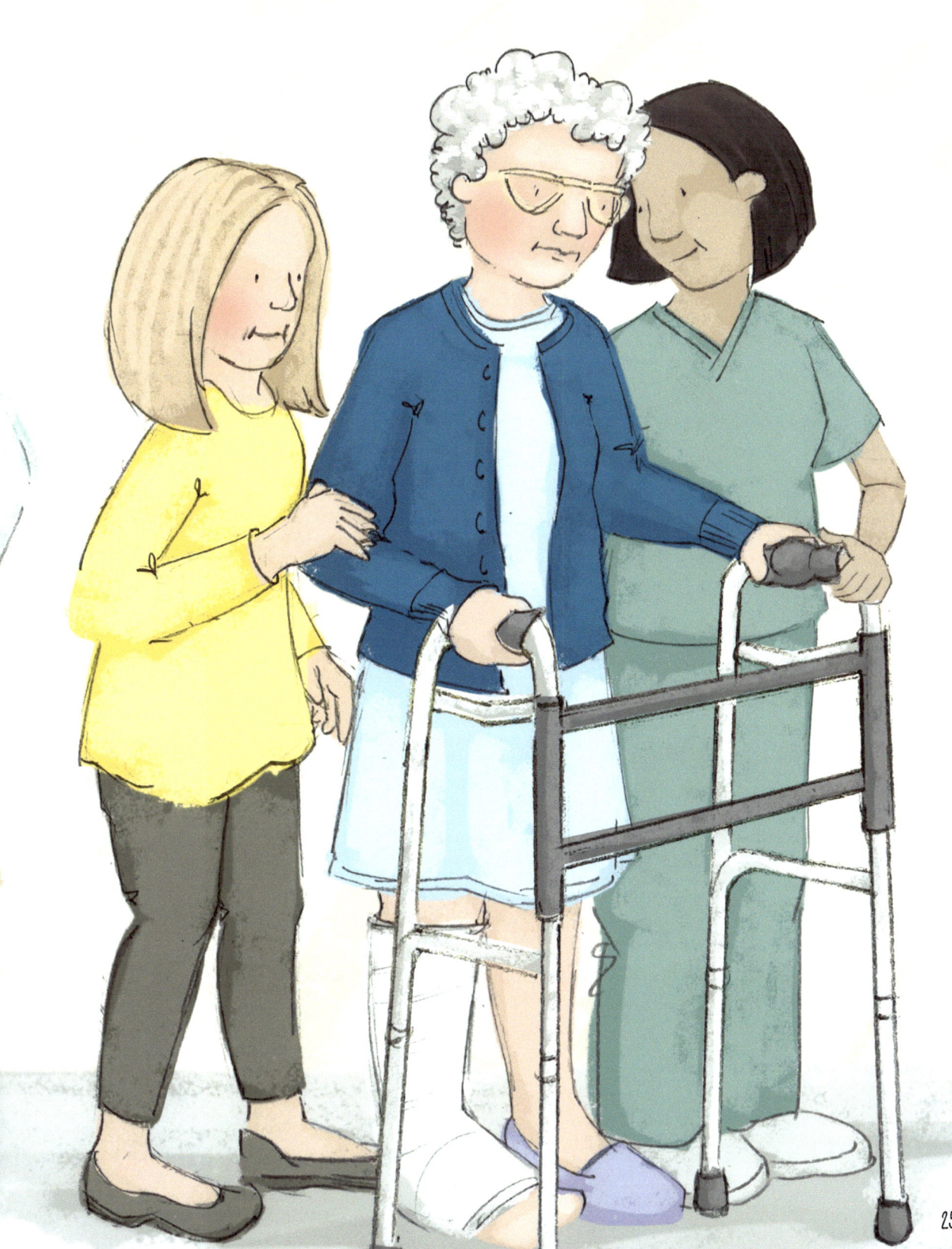

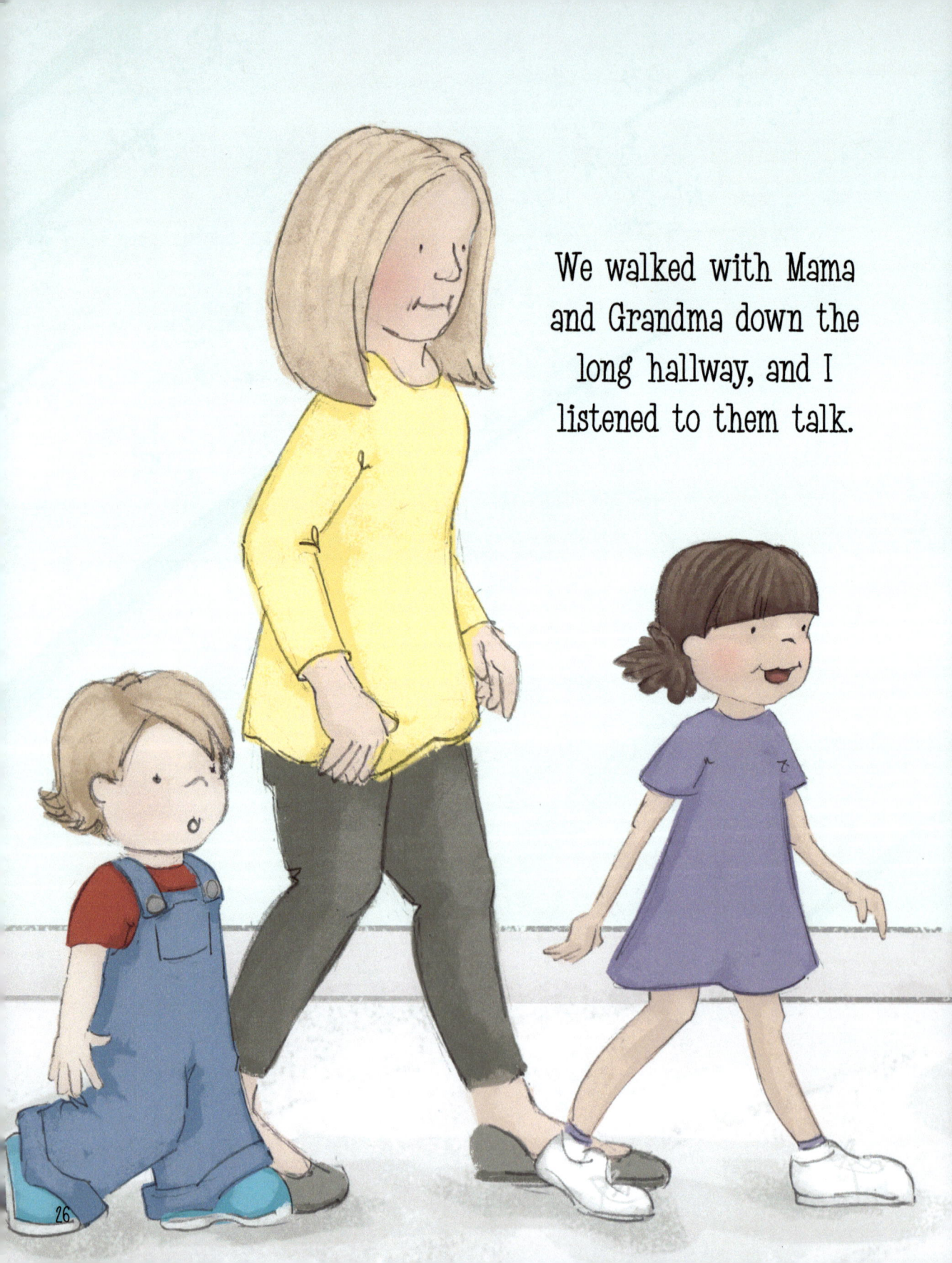

We walked with Mama and Grandma down the long hallway, and I listened to them talk.

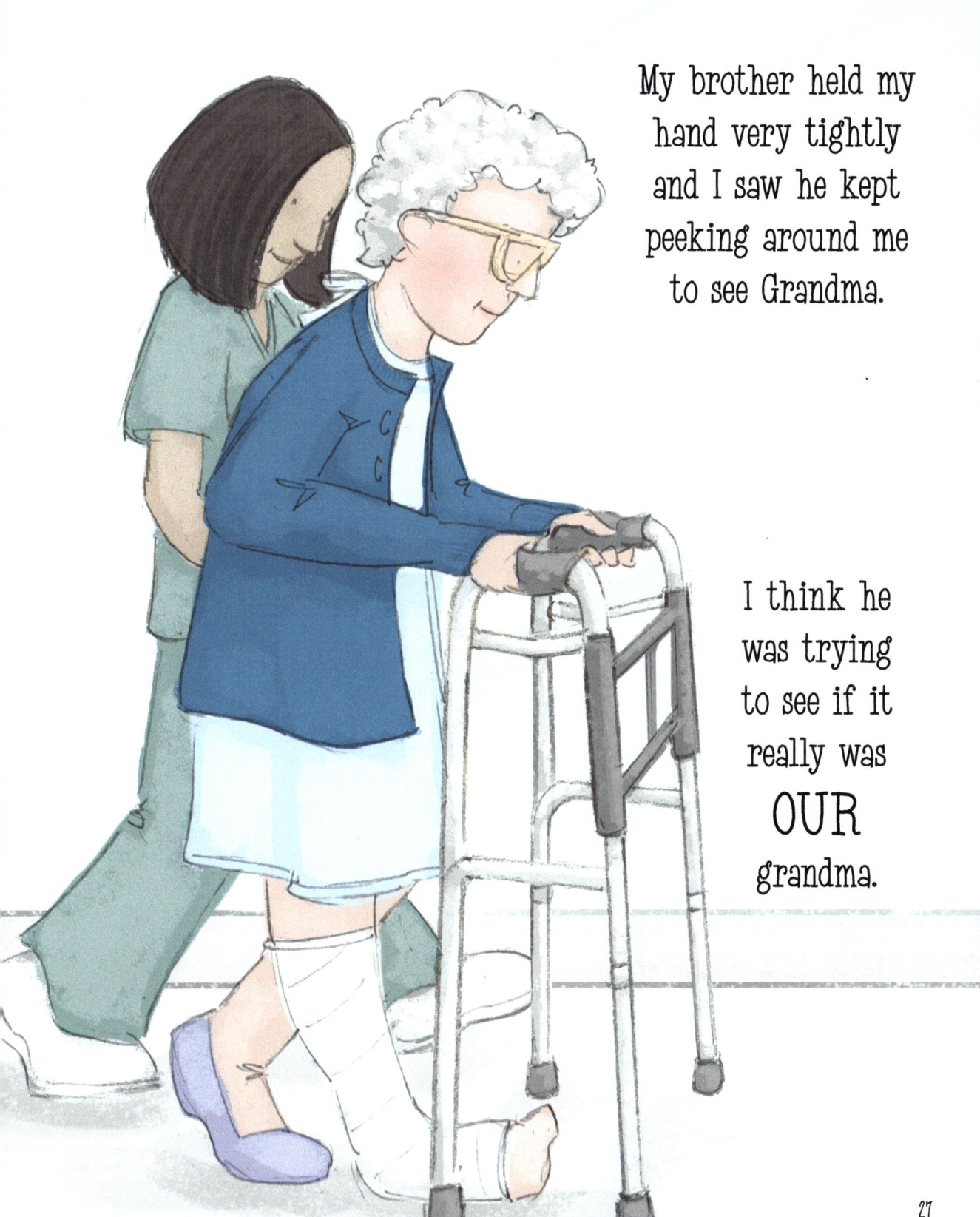

My brother held my hand very tightly and I saw he kept peeking around me to see Grandma.

I think he was trying to see if it really was OUR grandma.

When we got back to her room after a while, Grandma sat in a chair. She held out her arms and I ran and gave her a big hug.

I love Grandma!

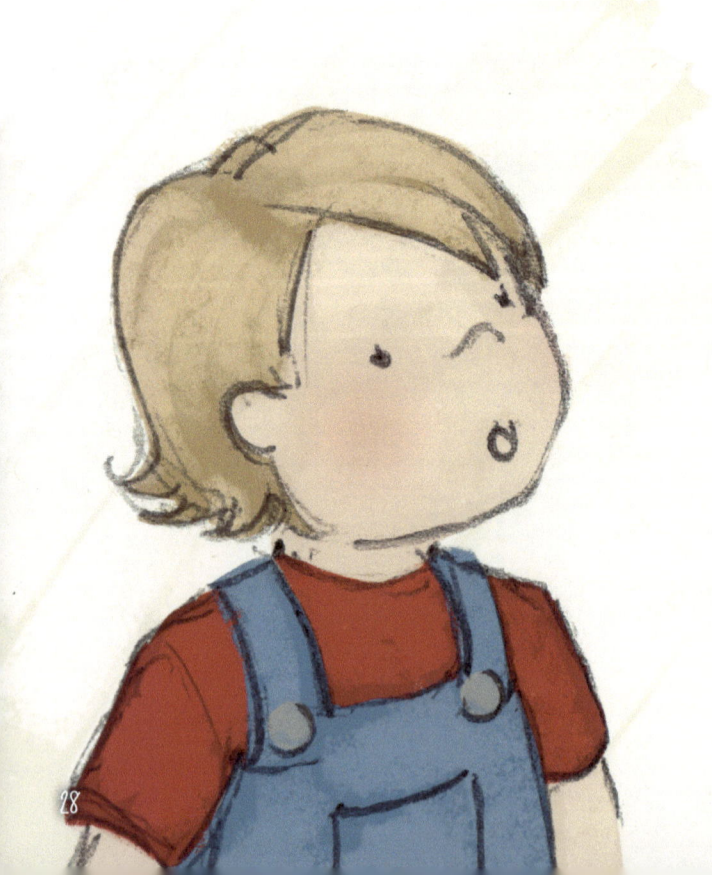

My brother came a little closer then.
He still didn't believe it was Grandma...

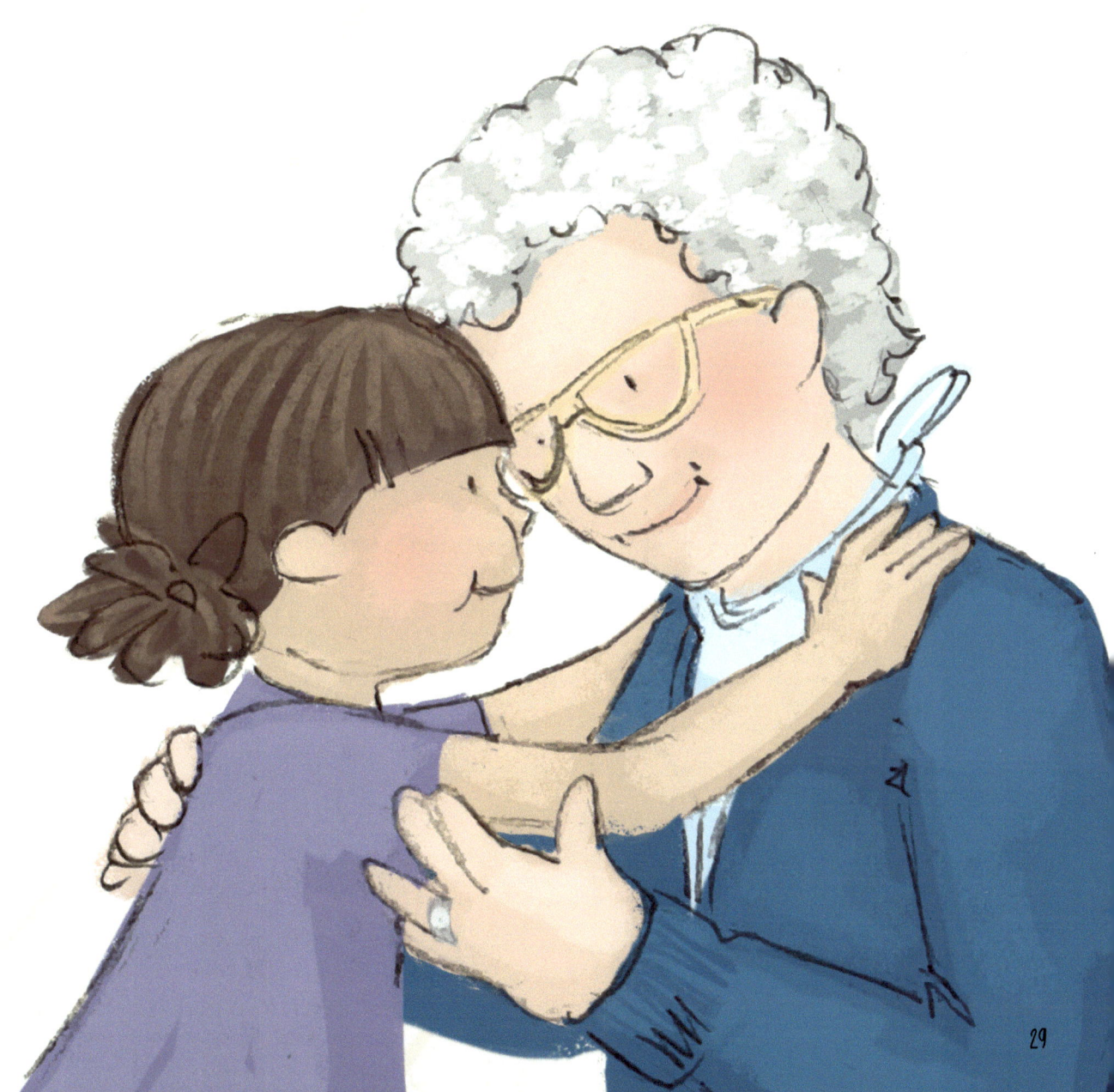

Then Grandma started talking about playing in the sandbox and jumping on the bed.

Suddenly my brother yelled, **"Grandma!"** and ran to give her a hug.

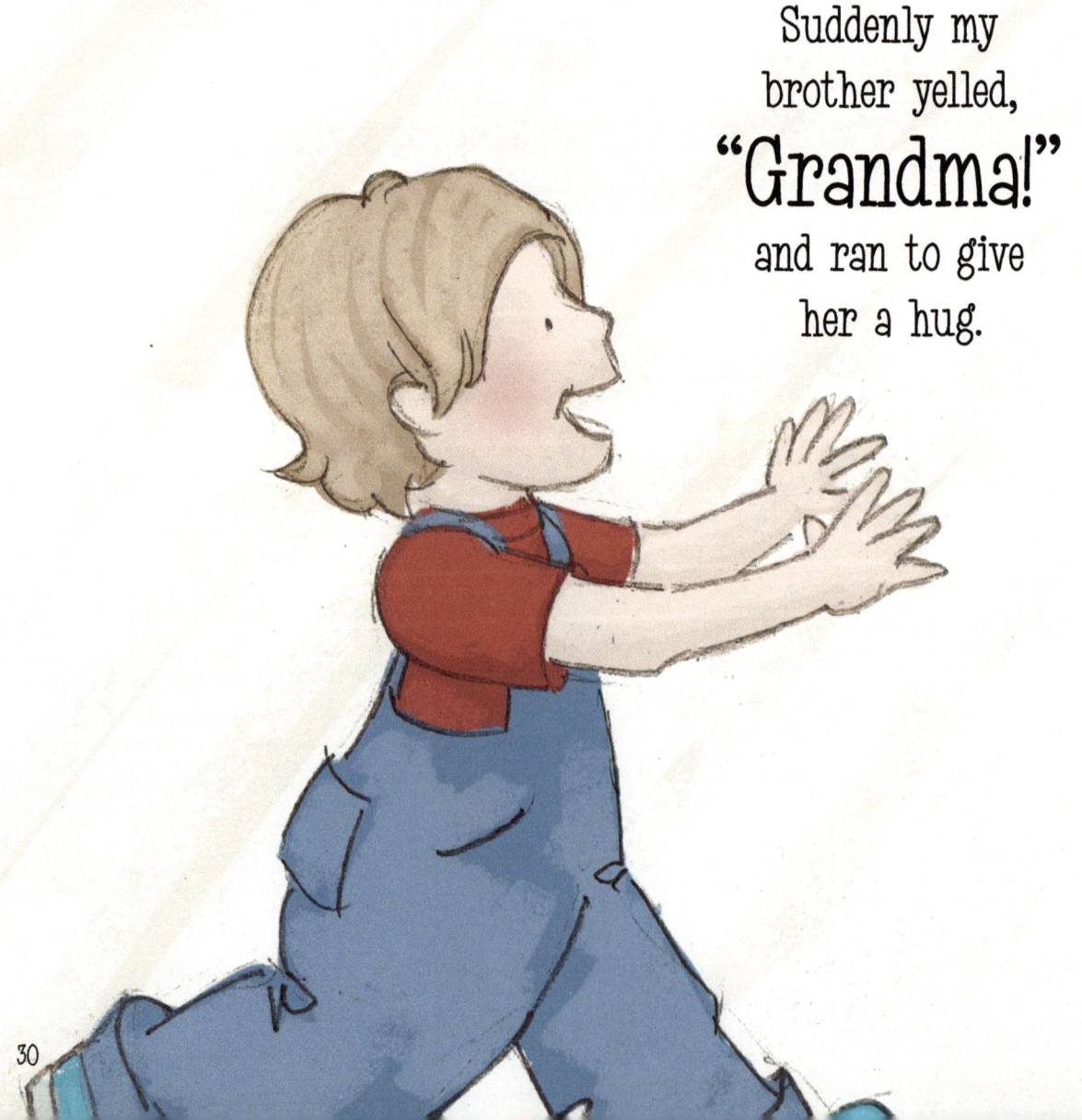

He sat in her lap and looked at me, smiling.

I nodded.

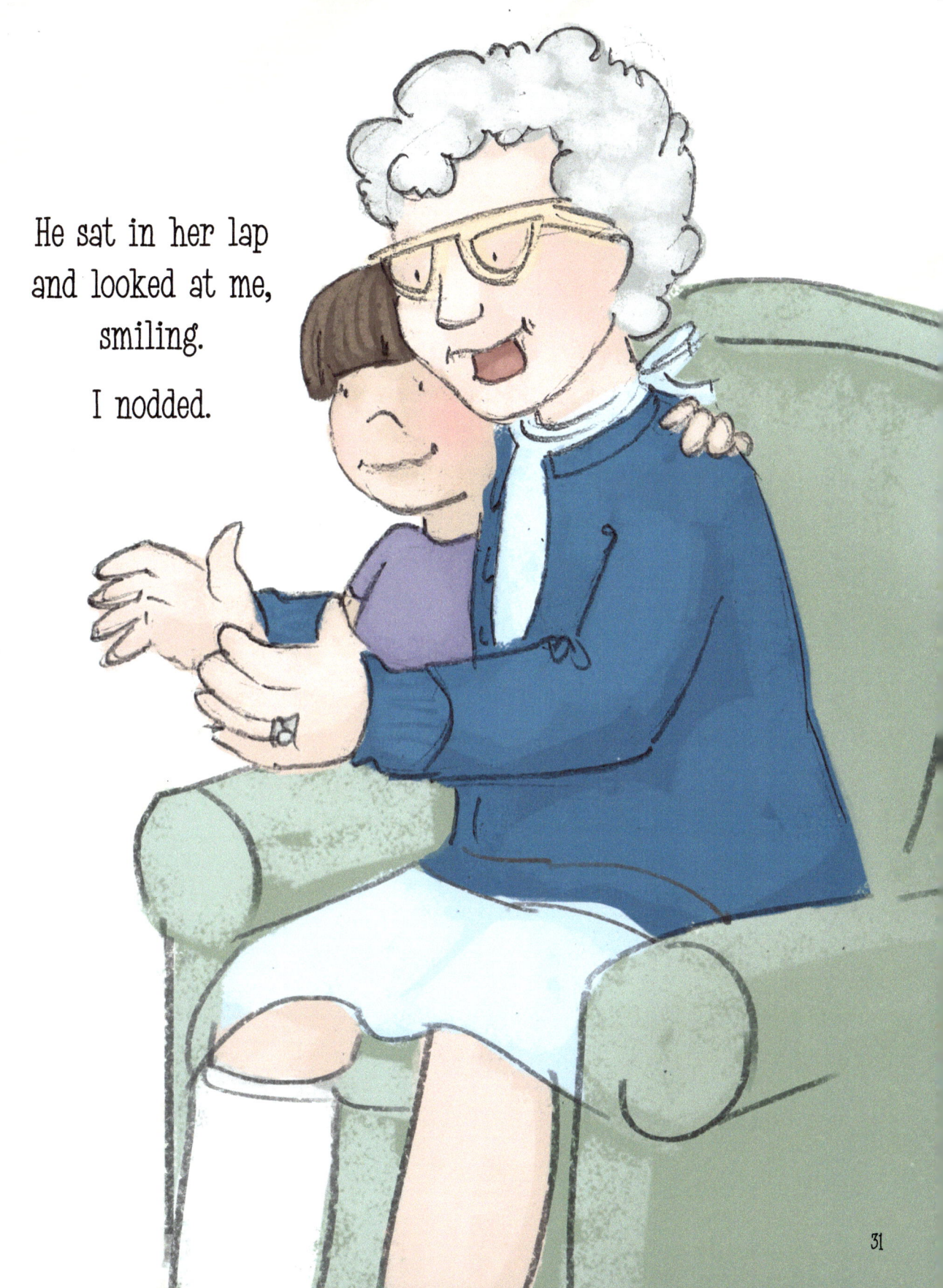

This IS our grandma!

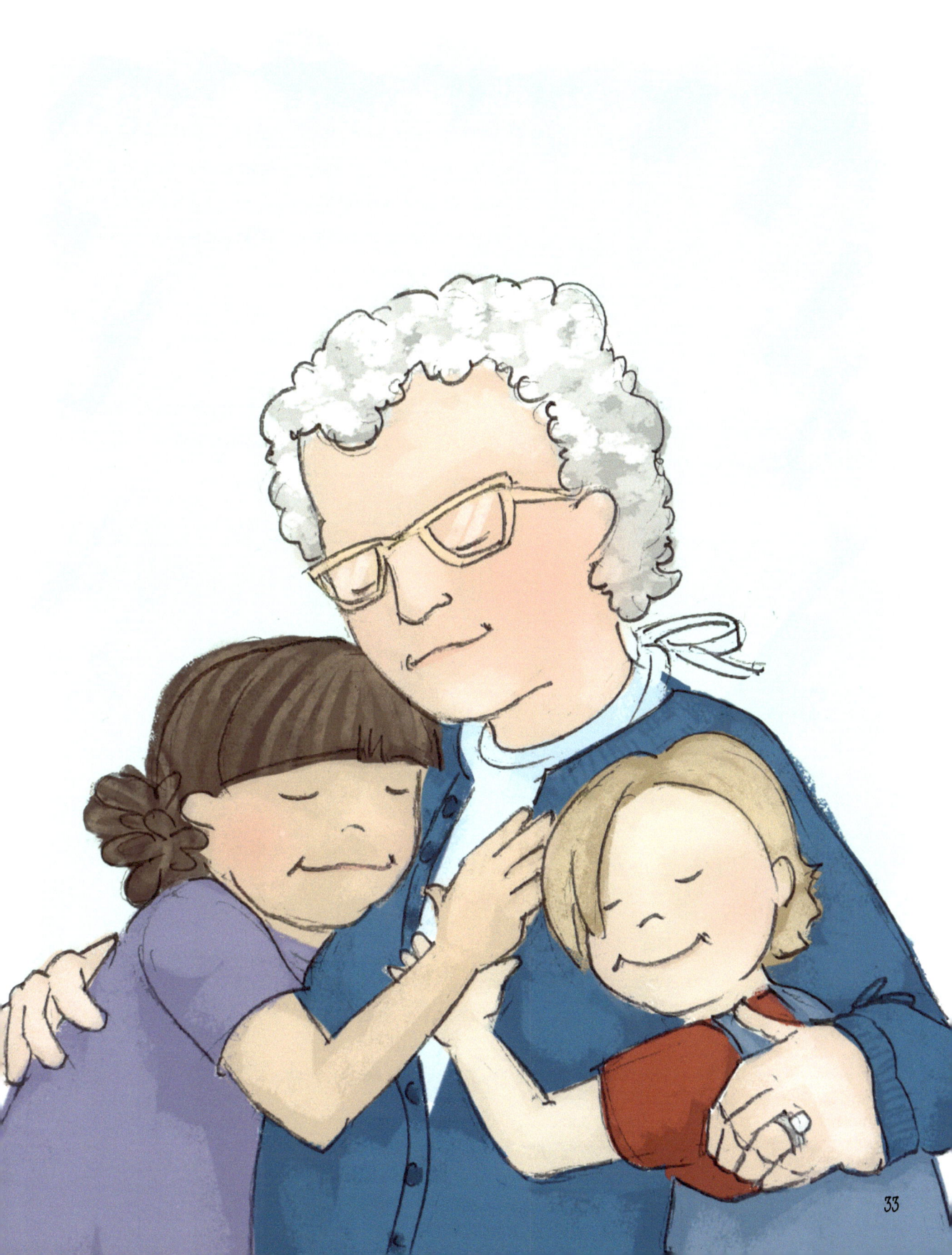

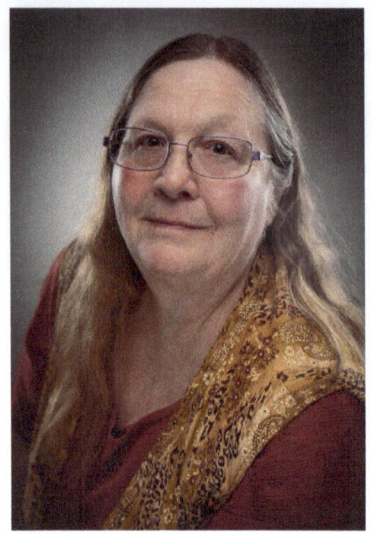

Paula Baysinger Morhardt

About the author

Paula Baysinger Morhardt lives in northwest Illinois with her two cats. When not writing, she spends her time gardening, cooking, and sewing. She also visits with her five grandchildren as much as possible. They especially enjoy watching wildlife together.

Is This My Grandma? is Paula's fourth children's book. Paula is the author of *Widow's Walk*, *Widow's Tears of Sorrow*, *Days of Daze*, *Night Maze*, *Sweet Sour Cherries*, *The Best Magic of All*, and *Through the Garden Window*, a series about gardening and cooking.

Also by Paula Baysinger Morhardt

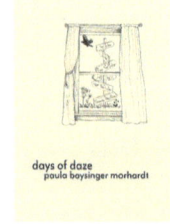

Days of Daze (2020)
POETRY CHAPBOOK
ISBN: 978-1-9525678-8-9

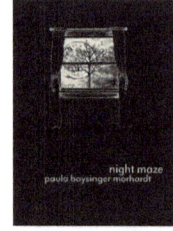

Night Maze (2020)
POETRY CHAPBOOK
ISBN: 978-1-9525670-1-8

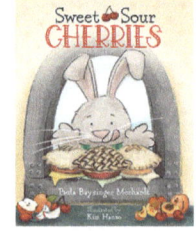

Sweet Sour Cherries (2020)
CHILDREN'S BOOK
ISBN: 978-1-952567-54-4 (hardcover)
ISBN: 978-1-952567-55-1 (softcover)

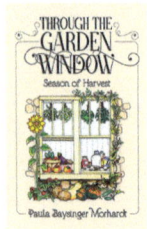

Through the Garden Window - Season of Harvest (2020)
1ST IN COOKBOOK SERIES
ISBN: 978-1-952567-58-2 (softcover spiral)

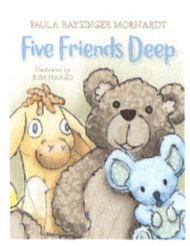

Five Friends Deep (2021)
CHILDREN'S BOOK
ISBN: 978-1-952567-64-3 (hardcover)
ISBN: 978-1-952567-65-0 (softcover)

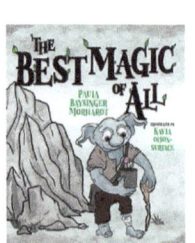

The Best Magic Of All (2021)
CHILDREN'S BOOK
ISBN: 978-1-952567-56-8 (hardcover)
ISBN: 978-1-952567-57-5 (softcover)

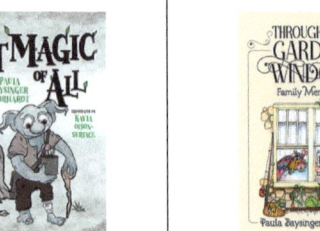

Through the Garden Window - Family Memories (2021)
2ND IN COOKBOOK SERIES
ISBN: 978-1-952567-59-9 (softcover spiral)

www.ingramcontent.com/pod-product-compliance
Lightning Source LLC
Chambersburg PA
CBHW041530070526
44586CB00002B/27